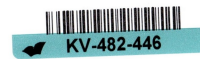

Modern Approach to Benign Esophageal Disease

Diagnosis and Surgical Therapy

Edited by

Cedric G. Bremner, M.B., B.Ch., Ch.M., F.R.C.S.(Eng), F.R.C.S.(Ed)

Professor of Clinical Surgery,
Department of Surgery, University of Southern California,
Los Angeles, California

Tom R. DeMeester, M.D.

Professor of Surgery and Chairman,
Department of Surgery, University of Southern California,
Los Angeles, California

Alberto Peracchia, M.D.

Professor of Surgery,
Department of General and Oncologic Surgery, University of Milan,
Milan, Italy

Quality Medical Publishing, Inc.

ST. LOUIS, MISSOURI
1995

PUBLISHER   Karen Berger
PROJECT MANAGER   Katherine Spakowski
PRODUCTION   Karen Kierath, Judy Bamert
BOOK DESIGN   Susan Trail
COVER DESIGN   Diane M. Beasley

Quality Medical Publishing, Inc.
11970 Borman Drive, Suite 222
St. Louis, Missouri 63146

ISBN 0-942219-96-1

VT/IPC/IPC   5   4   3   2   1

Modern Approach to
Benign Esophageal Disease

Diagnosis and Surgical Therapy

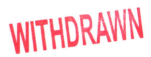

Contributors

Ermanno Ancona, M.D.
Professor of Surgery and Chairman,
Department of Surgery, University of Padua
School of Medicine, Padua, Italy

Marco Anselmino, M.D.
Department of Surgery, University of Padua
School of Medicine, Padua, Italy

Anthony Barlow, F.R.C.S.
Department of Surgery, Lincoln County
Hospital, Lincoln, United Kingdom

Gabriele Bianchi Porro, M.D.
Department of Gastroenterology, L. Sacco
Hospital, Milan, Italy

Luigi Bonavina, M.D.
Assistant Professor of Surgery, Department of
General and Oncologic Surgery, University of
Milan, Milan, Italy

Geoffrey W.B. Clark, F.R.C.S.(Ed)
Research Fellow, Department of Surgery,
University of Southern California, Los
Angeles, California

Mario Costantini, M.D.
Assistant Professor of Surgery, Department of
Surgery, University of Padua School of
Medicine, Padua, Italy

Peter F. Crookes, M.D.
Assistant Professor of Surgery, Department of
Surgery, University of Southern California, Los
Angeles, California

Tom R. DeMeester, M.D.
Professor of Surgery and Chairman,
Department of Surgery, University of Southern
California, Los Angeles, California

André Duranceau, M.D.
Professor of Surgery, Department of Surgery,
Division of Thoracic Surgery, University of
Montreal, Montreal, Quebec, Canada

Ernst Eypasch, M.D.
Department of Surgery, University of Cologne,
Cologne, Germany

Martin Fein, M.D.
Department of Surgery, Würzburg University
Hospital, Würzburg, Germany

Stephan M. Freys, M.D.
Department of Surgery, Würzburg University
Hospital, Würzburg, Germany

Karl H. Fuchs, M.D.
Professor of Surgery, Department of Surgery,
Würzburg University Hospital, Würzburg,
Germany

Jeffrey A. Hagen, M.D.
Assistant Professor of Surgery, Division of
Cardiothoracic Surgery, Department of
Surgery, University of Southern California, Los
Angeles, California

Johannes Heimbucher, M.D.
Department of Surgery, Würzburg University
Hospital, Würzburg, Germany

Raffaello Incarbone, M.D.
Department of General and Oncologic
Surgery, University of Milan, Milan, Italy

Werner K.H. Kauer, M.D.
Research Fellow, Department of Surgery,
University of Southern California, Los
Angeles, California

Owen Korn, M.D.
Department of Surgery, Technical University of Munich, Munich, Germany

Simon Y.K. Law, F.R.C.S.(Ed)
Research Fellow, Department of Surgery, University of Southern California, Los Angeles, California

Fabrizio Parente, M.D.
Department of Gastroenterology, L. Sacco Hospital, Milan, Italy

Alberto Peracchia, M.D.
Professor of Surgery, Department of General and Oncologic Surgery, University of Milan, Milan, Italy

Jeffrey H. Peters, M.D.
Assistant Professor of Surgery, Department of Surgery, University of Southern California, and Chief, Division of General Surgery, USC University Hospital, Los Angeles, California

Nancy Claire Poirier, M.D.
Department of Surgery, Division of Thoracic Surgery, University of Montreal, Montreal, Quebec, Canada

Manfred P. Ritter, M.D.
Research Fellow, Department of Surgery, University of Southern California, Los Angeles, California

Riccardo Rosati, M.D.
Assistant Professor of Surgery, Department of General and Oncologic Surgery, University of Milan, Milan, Italy

Andrea Segalin, M.D.
Assistant Professor of Surgery, Department of General and Oncologic Surgery, University of Milan, Milan, Italy

Hubert J. Stein, M.D.
Department of Surgery, Technical University of Munich, Munich, Germany

Raymond Taillefer, M.D.
Department of Surgery, Division of Thoracic Surgery, University of Montreal, Montreal, Quebec, Canada

Hartmut Thomas, M.D.
Department of Surgery, Greifswald University, Greifswald, Germany

Thomas J. Watson, M.D.
Clinical Instructor in Surgery, Department of Surgery, University of Southern California, Los Angeles, California

Giovanni Zaninotto, M.D.
Assistant Professor of Surgery, Department of Surgery, University of Padua School of Medicine, Padua, Italy

Preface

Interest in benign esophageal disease is undergoing a revival among surgeons. Factors fostering this renewed interest include the emergence of focused interest in an ever-expanding knowledge base of general surgery, the availability of modern technology that allows testing of foregut function in an ambulatory office setting, and the reduced morbidity and greater patient acceptance of surgical therapy through limited access technology.

The outgrowth of this interest has been the development of a new brand of modern surgeons. They are characterized as having a disease focus as opposed to a focus on the procedure. They understand and are skilled in the diagnosis of disease by the measurement of altered organ function rather than by the presence of an anatomic lesion. They apply surgical therapy to improve the function of an organ by altering its structure or the arrangement of its moving parts rather than extirpation of the organ. While being talented open surgeons, they have become adept in the use of the new tools of limited access surgery.

The authors of the chapters contained in this book are among such modern surgeons. In common, they have passed through our laboratories or clinical services during the acquirement of their knowledge and skills. The focus of this book is the physiologic approach to the understanding and management of esophageal disease. This is coupled with the utilization of minimally invasive thoracoscopic and laparoscopic surgery as a first option in the treatment of gastroesophageal reflux disease, esophageal motility disorders, esophageal diverticula, and benign esophageal tumors. Open surgery is reserved for the initial approach to complicated esophageal disease, reoperation of previously failed procedures, or esophageal replacement for end-stage benign disease. As such the contributions report the present status of a changing approach to the exciting field of esophageal surgery. In so doing, these authors have emerged as our critics and moved the science of esophageal surgery forward.

Tom R. DeMeester, M.D.
Alberto Peracchia, M.D.
Cedric G. Bremner, M.B., Ch.M.

This publication
was made possible by
a generous educational grant
from

The Ethicon Foundation

Contents

1

Pathophysiology of Esophageal Motor Disorders and Gastroesophageal Reflux Disease

Hubert J. Stein, M.D. • *Owen Korn, M.D.*

The esophagus of the adult human is a 24 to 27 cm long muscular tube with tonically contracted sphincters at the oral and aboral end. Its function can be visualized mechanically as a worm-drive pump with a one-way valve at each end. The valves act as barriers separating compartments with different baseline pressures (Fig. 1-1). A coordinated interplay between the pump of the esophageal body and the adjacent valves is essential to propel food from the mouth to the stomach and prevent reflux of gastric contents. Failure of the propulsive ability of the esophageal

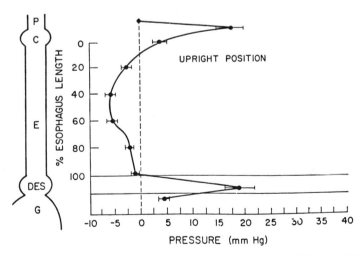

Fig. 1-1 Resting pressure profile of the foregut showing the pressure differential between the atmospheric pharyngeal pressure *(P)*, the less-than-atmospheric midesophageal pressure *(E)*, and the greater-than-atmospheric intragastric pressure *(G)*, with the interposed high pressure zones of the cricopharyngeus *(C)* and distal esophageal sphincter *(DES)*. (From Waters PF, DeMeester TR. Foregut motor disorders and their surgical management. Med Clin North Am 65:1237-1272, 1981.)

body or uncoordinated relaxation of the proximal and distal valve hampers the forward movement of food. A compromised resistance of the distal valve promotes reflux of gastric contents.

Nonobstructive dysphagia, that is, dysphagia in the absence of structural abnormalities, is the primary symptom of a disturbed propulsion through the esophagus, whereas heartburn and regurgitation are usually ascribed to excessive reflux of gastric contents. However, symptoms alone are not a good indicator for the presence and type of disorder because esophageal motor disorders, gastroesophageal reflux, and extraesophageal disorders may cause indistinguishable symptoms. In addition, the perception of a symptom by the patient is a balance between the severity of the underlying abnormality and the patient's adjustment to that difficulty. Consequently, any complaint of dysphagia, heartburn, or regurgitation requires a detailed assessment of the patient's dietary history in addition to a clear understanding of the normal physiology and pathophysiology mechanisms that may cause a disturbance in the normal action of the esophagus and its adjacent valves.[1,2]

PHYSIOLOGY OF ESOPHAGEAL FUNCTION

The act of swallowing consists of the oral, pharyngeal, and esophageal phases. During the oral phase of swallowing, food is taken into the mouth and chewed into a variety of bite sizes. When food is ready for swallowing, the tongue, acting like a piston, moves the bolus into the posterior oropharynx and forces it into the hypopharynx. This phase of swallowing is completely under conscious control.

With arrival of food in the oropharynx, a complex reflex pattern is initiated that controls the pharyngeal phase of swallowing. This is triggered by sensory nerve endings located in the anterior and posterior tonsillar pillars and the posterior lateral walls of the hypopharynx. The afferent nerves of the pharynx are the glossopharyngeal nerve and the superior laryngeal branches of the vagus. Once aroused by stimuli entering via these nerves, the swallowing center in the medulla coordinates the complete act of swallowing by discharging impulses through the fifth, seventh, tenth, eleventh, and twelfth cranial nerves, as well as the motor neurons of C1 to C3. Discharges through these nerves occur in a rather specific pattern and last for approximately 0.5 second. During this phase the soft palate is elevated to separate the oropharynx from the nasopharynx. This prevents pressure generated in the oropharynx from being dissipated through the nose. The hyoid bone moves upward and anteriorly, elevating the larynx and opening the retrolaryngeal space. The epiglottis tilts backward, thus covering the opening of the larynx and deflecting the swallowed bolus posteriorly and laterally. Respiration is reflexly inhibited to prevent aspiration. Simultaneously the bolus is pushed through the pharynx by a strong peristaltic contraction. The whole pharyngeal phase of swallowing occurs within 1.5 seconds.

The esophageal phase of swallowing begins with the relaxation of the cricopharyngeus or upper esophageal sphincter. In the normal situation this occurs in coordination with the pharyngeal contraction. The pressure gradient between the pharyngeal pressure and the less-than-atmospheric midesophageal or intrathoracic pressure (Fig. 1-1) speeds the movement of food from the hypopharynx into the esophagus when the cricopharyngeus relaxes. The bolus is both propelled by the peristaltic contractions of the posterior laryngeal constrictors and sucked into the thoracic esophagus. The compliance of the cervical esophagus is critical for this phase of swallowing. The upper esophageal sphincter closes within another 0.5 second, with the immediate closing pressure reaching approximately twice the resting level. This postrelaxation contraction continues down the esophagus as a peristaltic wave (Fig. 1-2). The high closing pressure and the initiation of the peristaltic wave prevent regurgitation of the bolus from the esophagus back into the pharynx. After the peristaltic wave has passed further down the esophagus, the pressure in the upper esophageal sphincter returns to its resting level (Fig. 1-2).

The striated muscles of the cricopharyngeus and the upper third of the esophagus are activated by efferent fibers distributed through the vagus nerves and its recurrent laryngeal branches. The integrity of innervation is required for the cricopharyngeus to relax in coordination with the pharyngeal contraction and resume its resting tone once a bolus has entered the upper esophagus.

The body of the esophagus functions as a worm-drive propulsive pump, because of the helical arrangement of its circular muscles, and is responsible for trans-

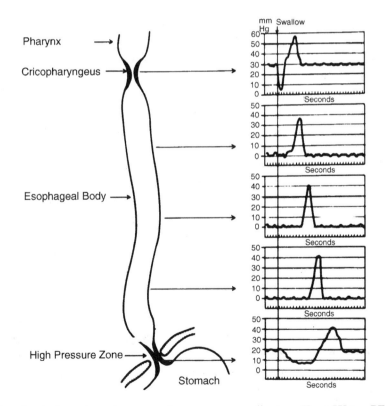

Fig. 1-2 Intraluminal esophageal pressures in response to swallowing. (From Waters PF, DeMeester TR. Foregut motor disorders and their surgical management. Med Clin North Am 65:1237-1272, 1981.)

mitting a food bolus from the distal esophagus into the stomach. This phase of swallowing represents esophageal work done during alimentation. Food is moved into the stomach from a pressure of −6 mm Hg intrathoracic pressure to an average of 6 mm Hg intra-abdominal pressure, a gradient of 12 mm Hg (Fig. 1-1). Effective and coordinated smooth muscle function in the lower third of the esophagus is therefore important in pumping the food into the stomach. The peristaltic wave generates an occlusive pressure varying from 30 to 150 mm Hg (Fig. 1-2). The wave rises to a peak in 1 second, lasts at the peak for approximately 0.5 second, and then subsides in approximately 1.5 seconds. The peak of a primary peristaltic wave, a peristaltic contraction sequence initiated by a pharyngeal swallow, moves down the esophagus at 2 to 4 cm/sec and reaches the distal esophagus approximately 9 seconds after swallowing has been initiated (Fig. 1-2). Consecutive swallows produce similar primary peristaltic waves, but when the act of swallowing is rapidly repeated, the esophagus remains relaxed and the peristaltic wave occurs only after the last movement of the pharynx. This phenomenon is referred to as "postdeglutitive inhibition." Orderly contractions of the muscular wall and anchoring of the esophagus at its inferior end are necessary for efficient and aboral propulsion to occur.

Progress of the wave in the esophagus is caused by sequential activation of its muscles initiated by efferent vagal nerve fibers arising in the swallowing center. Continuity of the esophageal muscle is not necessary if the nerves are intact. If the muscles but not the nerves are cut, the pressure wave begins distally below the cut and dies out at the proximal end above the cut. This allows a sleeve resection of the esophagus to be done without destroying its normal function. Afferent impulses from receptors within the esophageal wall are not essential for progress of the coordinated wave. However, if the esophagus is distended at any point, a contractual wave begins with a forceful closure of the upper esophageal sphincter and sweeps down the esophagus. This secondary peristalsis occurs without any movements of the mouth or pharynx. Secondary contractions can occur as an independent local reflex to clear the esophagus of material left behind after the passage of the primary wave but are less common than previously thought.

The lower esophageal sphincter in humans is a unique one-way valve that separates the stomach with its positive pressure environment from the negative pressure environment in the chest (Fig. 1-1). In the normal situation the sphincter actively remains closed to prevent reflux of gastric contents into the esophagus and opens temporarily by relaxation to permit passage of food from the esophagus into the stomach. This relaxation coincides with a pharyngeal swallow (Fig. 1-2). The lower esophageal sphincter pressure returns to its resting level after the peristaltic wave has passed through the esophagus. Consequently, reflux of gastric juice that may occur through the open valve during a swallow is pumped back into the stomach. If the pharyngeal swallow does not initiate a peristaltic contraction, the coincident relaxation of the lower esophageal sphincter is unguarded and reflux of gastric juice can occur. This appears to be the major cause of the so-called transient or spontaneous lower esophageal sphincter relaxations.

Despite the clear manometric findings of a high pressure zone in the distal esophagus, the existence and structural equivalent of the lower esophageal sphinc-

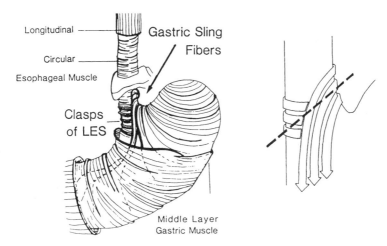

Fig. 1-3 Orientation of muscle fibers at the gastroesophageal junction and their mode of action shown schematically. LES = lower esophageal sphincter. (Modified from Liebermann-Meffert D, Allgower M, Schmid P, et al. Muscular equivalent of the esophageal sphincter. Gastroenterology 76:31-38, 1979.)

ter in humans has been a matter of speculation for many years.[3,4] Anatomic studies have shown that in humans there is no circular or annular muscle at the gastroesophageal junction. The assessment of fiber specimen shows that the muscle bundles of the external longitudinal layer run straight down the esophagus to pass the junction with the stomach. The much shorter bundles of the internal muscular sheath take their course perpendicularly to the external layer and form incomplete circles around the esophageal lumen. These semicircles diverge abruptly at the level of the gastroesophageal junction into long and short bundles with opposite orientation. One part, the so-called gastric "sling," hooks around the gastric fundus, forms the cardiac notch, and embraces the anterior and posterior walls of the stomach. The other parts, the so-called semicircular "clasps," retain their orientation and hook around the lesser curvature (Fig. 1-3).

Microdissection studies show that the muscular fibers of both the gastric "sling" and the "clasps" increase in number and concentration across the gastroesophageal junction and become superimposed on each other. This results in a two- to threefold asymmetric thickening of the inner muscular layer that is maximal at the gastroesophageal junction and is most prominent and longest at the cardiac notch toward the greater curvature side (Fig. 1-4, *left*). Although significant, this asymmetric thickening of the muscular structures does not form a mass that can be easily palpated. The asymmetric muscular thickening at the gastroesophageal junction is, however, mirrored in the manometric asymmetry of the lower esophageal high pressure zone (Fig. 1-4, *center* and *right*). Both the area of greatest muscle thickness and the highest manometric sphincter pressures correlate with the location of the so-called gastric "sling" fibers. The finding that the cholinergic response of the lower esophageal sphincter has regional variations, together with these anatomic

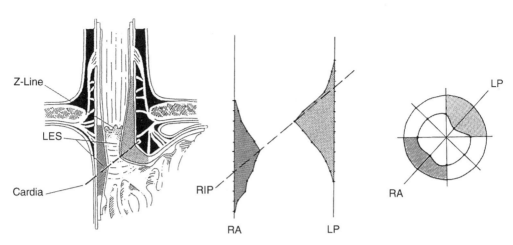

Fig. 1-4 Muscle thickness and radial manometric pressures at the gastroesophageal junction in humans. *Left:* Muscle thickness at the lesser and greater curvature. *Center:* Manometric pressures along the gastroesophageal junction at the lesser and greater curvature side of the stomach. *Right:* Radial manometric pressures at the respiratory inversion point. LES = lower esophageal sphincter; RID = respiratory inversion point; RA = right anterior; LP = left posterior. (Based on data by Stein HJ, Lieberman-Meffert D, DeMeester TR, et al. Three-dimensional pressure image and muscular structure of the human lower esophageal sphincter. Surgery 1995 [in press].)

and manometric observations, suggests that the manometric lower esophageal sphincter in humans has two distinct functional muscle units at the gastroesophageal junction: the gastric "sling" at the cardiac notch and the semicircular "clasps" on the lesser curvature side.[5]

PATHOPHYSIOLOGIC ASPECTS OF ESOPHAGEAL FUNCTION

Disorders of the coordinated interplay between the various phases of swallowing are clinically best classified into disorders of the pharyngoesophageal phase of swallowing, primary motor disorders of the esophageal body, lower esophageal sphincter disorders associated with gastroesophageal reflux disease, and the so-called secondary esophageal motor disorders.

Pharyngoesophageal Motor Disorders

Disorders of the pharyngoesophageal phase of swallowing result from an incoordination of the neuromuscular events involved in chewing, initiation of swallowing, and propulsion of the material from the oropharynx to the cervical esophagus. This results in dysphagia, pharyngeal regurgitation, aspiration, and repetitive respiratory infections. The mechanisms responsible for pharyngoesophageal dysfunction include (1) inadequate oropharyngeal bolus transport; (2) inability to pressurize the pharynx; (3) inability to elevate the larynx; (4) incoordination of cricopharyngeal relaxation and pharyngeal contraction; and (5) decreased compliance of the pharyngoesophageal segment secondary to a restrictive myopathy.

Pharyngoesophageal swallowing disorders are either congenital or acquired and involve the central and peripheral nervous systems. They include cerebrovascular accidents, brain stem tumors, poliomyelitis, multiple sclerosis, Parkinson's disease, pseudobulbar palsy, peripheral neuropathy, or operative damage to the cranial nerves involved in swallowing. Muscular diseases such as radiation-induced myopathy, dermatomyositis, myotonic dystrophy, and myasthenia gravis are less common. Occasionally, extrinsic compression by thyromegaly, cervical lymphadenopathy, or hyperostosis of the cervical spine can cause cervical dysphagia.

The rapidity of the oropharyngeal phase of swallowing, the movement of the gullet, and the asymmetry of the cricopharyngeus account for the difficulty in assessing abnormalities of esophagopharyngeal swallowing disorders with conventional manometry. Video/cine radiography is currently the most useful objective test to evaluate oropharyngeal bolus transport, pharyngeal contraction, cricopharyngeal relaxation, and the dynamics of airway protection during swallowing.[2] Careful analysis of video/cine radiographic studies and manometry using specially designed catheters, ideally performed simultaneously, can identify the cause of pharyngoesophageal dysfunction in most situations.

It has been difficult to consistently demonstrate a motility abnormality of the pharyngoesophageal segment in patients with Zenker's diverticulum. The abnormality most likely to be present is a loss of compliance of the pharyngoesophageal segment manifested by an increased bolus pressure.[6] Esophageal muscle biopsies in patients with Zenker's diverticulum have shown histologic evidence of a fibrotic myopathy, which correlates with a decreased compliance of the upper esophagus on video/cine radiographic and detailed manometric studies. These findings suggest that the diverticulum develops as a consequence of the repetitive stress of bolus transport through a noncompliant muscle of the pharyngoesophageal segment. Other manifestations of a noncompliant segment in the proximal esophagus are a cricopharyngeal bar or more extended narrowing of the pharyngoesophageal segment.

Incoordination of the sphincter relaxation with pharyngeal contraction is another cause for the development of Zenker's diverticulum. This may not occur throughout the full length of the sphincter and can easily be missed on manometric assessment because of movement of the cricopharyngeus on swallowing. Failure of the cricopharyngeal muscle to relax on swallowing and failure of an esophageal contraction after a pharyngeal swallow have also been observed in patients with Zenker's diverticulum.[7]

Primary Esophageal Motor Disorders

Motor abnormalities in the worm-drive pump of the esophageal body or the lower esophageal sphincter can give rise to a number of disorders that usually result in dysphagia and/or regurgitation. These symptoms may be due to a nonrelaxing lower esophageal sphincter, disorganized contractions of the esophageal body, or a combination of both. Animal studies and some clinical evidence indicate that the function of the esophageal body can deteriorate secondary to distal obstruction and may recover if the obstruction is relieved early during the disease process.

With the introduction of standard esophageal manometry, a number of primary esophageal motility disorders have been classified as separate disease entities. These include achalasia, diffuse esophageal spasm, the so-called "nutcracker esophagus," and the hypertensive lower esophageal sphincter[8,9] (Table 1-1).

The classification of these disorders is usually based on the analysis of the manometric recordings of only a few wet swallows performed in a laboratory setting. The recently introduced technique of ambulatory 24-hour monitoring of esophageal motor activity multiplies the number of esophageal contractions available for analysis and provides an opportunity to assess esophageal motor function under a variety of physiologic situations. This increases the accuracy and dependability of the measurement.[10] Ambulatory 24-hour esophageal motility monitoring has demonstrated that there are marked differences in the classification of esopha-

Table 1-1 Classification and manometric characteristics of the primary esophageal motor disorders

Achalasia

Incomplete lower esophageal sphincter relaxation
Aperistalsis of the esophageal body
Elevated lower esophageal sphincter pressure
Increased intraesophageal baseline pressures

Diffuse esophageal spasm

Frequent simultaneous contractions
Intermittent normal peristalsis
Repetitive and multipeaked contractions
Contractions of increased amplitude and duration

Nutcracker esophagus

Increased mean peristaltic amplitude in the distal esophagus
Increased mean duration of contractions
Normal peristaltic sequence

Hypertensive lower esophageal sphincter

Elevated lower esophageal sphincter pressure
Normal lower esophageal sphincter relaxation
Normal peristalsis of the esophageal body

Nonspecific esophageal motility disorders

Decreased or absent amplitude of esophageal peristalsis
Increased number of nontransmitted contractions
Abnormal waveforms
Normal lower esophageal sphincter pressure and relaxation

geal motor disorders when compared to standard manometry techniques (Fig. 1-5). The degree of reclassification of esophageal motor disorders resulting from analysis of ambulatory manometry studies indicates that the classification of esophageal motor disorders based on standard manometry is inappropriate. The intermittency of esophageal motor abnormalities can be missed easily or overdiagnosed in the unphysiologic setting of standard manometry, but are detected with a higher degree of reliability when motor activity is monitored over 24 hours in a variety of physiologic conditions. Based on these observations, esophageal motility disorders should be viewed as a spectrum of abnormalities that reflect various stages of destruction of esophageal motor function rather than separate entities.

Using simultaneous manometry and fluoroscopy, Kahrilas et al.[11] documented that esophageal contraction sequences that are not propulsive, and that do not have a minimum amplitude of 30 mm Hg, are not able to propel a bolus through the esophagus. This correlates with the observation that patients with nonobstructive dysphagia show an inability of the esophageal body to organize the motor activity into peristaltic contractions during meals. In normal asymptomatic volunteers the prevalence of "effective contractions," peristaltic contractions with sufficient amplitude to propel a bolus, increases with increasing states of consciousness, that is, from sleep, to upright, and to meal periods. This is probably due to a modulatory effect of the central nervous system on esophageal motor activity. Patients with nonobstructive dysphagia lack this ability to increase the prevalence of "effective contractions" with increasing states of consciousness. The frequency of "effective contractions" during meal periods thus allows an expression of the severity of

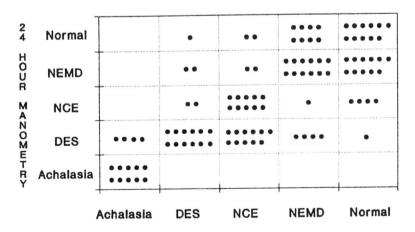

Fig. 1-5 Classification of esophageal motor disorders in 108 patients with dysphagia and/or noncardiac chest pain according to the findings on standard or ambulatory 24-hour manometry. DES = diffuse esophageal spasm; NCE = nutcracker esophagus; NEMD = nonspecific esophageal motor disorder. (From Stein HJ, DeMeester TR, Eypasch EP, et al. Ambulatory 24-hour esophageal manometry in the evaluation of esophageal motor disorders and noncardiac chest pain. Surgery 110: 753-763, 1991.)

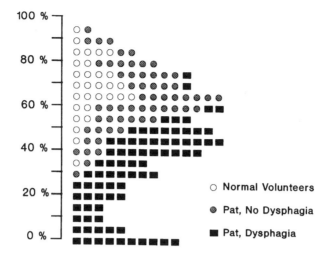

Fig. 1-6 Prevalence of "effective contractions" during meal periods in normal volunteers, patients with nonobstructive dysphagia, and patients without dysphagia. Less than 50% "effective contractions" during meals are associated with a high prevalence of nonobstructive dysphagia.

esophageal body dysfunction on a linear scale (Fig. 1-6). The use of this parameter for the evaluation of esophageal body function obviates the need for the current categories of esophageal motor disorders and permits an objective assessment of the effect of medical or surgical therapy.[12]

It has been suggested that esophageal contractions of abnormally high amplitude or long duration are responsible for chest pain in patients with esophageal motor disorders. Ambulatory 24-hour motility monitoring in these patients has, however, shown that chest pain is rarely related to abnormal esophageal motor activity. Rather, episodes of gastroesophageal reflux appear to be the most common esophageal cause of noncardiac chest pain. Occasionally a markedly increased frequency of simultaneous and repetitive contractions appears to precede chest pain.[13] Esophageal blood supply may be interrupted during these bursts of abnormal muscular contractions in a similar way to cardiac ischemia. The ischemia may become critical in situations where the resting blood flow to the esophagus is already compromised, as demonstrated in the hypertrophic esophageal muscle of patients with esophageal motor disorders. A burst of disorganized motor activity in this situation may give rise to ischemic pain. Consequently, we have termed chest pain caused by a burst of incoordinated esophageal motor activity under ischemic conditions "esophageal claudication."[13]

Gastroesophageal Reflux Disease

Gastroesophageal reflux disease (GERD) is the single most common foregut disorder and accounts for approximately 75% of esophageal pathology. The disease

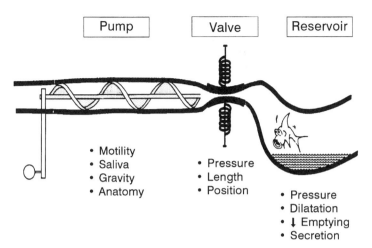

Fig. 1-7 Mechanical model of the esophagus as a propulsive pump, the lower esophageal sphincter as a valve, and the stomach as a reservoir. Esophageal clearance of refluxed gastric juice is determined by the esophageal motor activity, salivation, gravity, and the presence of an anatomic alteration such as a hiatal hernia. The competency of the lower esophageal sphincter depends on its pressure, overall length, and length exposed to abdominal pressure. Gastric function abnormalities causing gastroesophageal reflux include increased intragastric pressure, gastric dilation, decreased emptying rate, and increased gastric acid secretion. (From Stein HJ, DeMeester TR, Hinder RA. Outpatient physiologic testing and surgical management of foregut motility disorders. Curr Probl Surg 29:415-555, 1992.)

can be manifested by typical and atypical symptoms and leads to esophageal mucosal injury in approximately 50% of affected patients.[2] Despite its prevalence, the pathophysiologic factors leading to increased esophageal exposure to gastric contents and the development of mucosal injury have only recently emerged.

Increased esophageal exposure to gastric juice may result from three known causes. The first is a mechanically defective lower esophageal sphincter, which is present in approximately 60% to 70% of patients with GERD. The identification of a defective sphincter as the cause of increased esophageal acid exposure is important because it is the one causative factor that antireflux surgery is designed to correct. The other two causes are inefficient esophageal clearance of refluxed gastric juice and abnormalities of the gastric reservoir that augment physiologic reflux. These factors cannot be corrected by an antireflux procedure. Conceptually, the three main causes of gastroesophageal reflux can be thought of as the failure of a pump, a valve, or a reservoir (Fig. 1-7). The relative contributions of each of these components of the antireflux mechanism to increased esophageal exposure to gastric juice should be determined prior to considering specific therapy for the disease. The distribution of these causes of gastroesophageal reflux in a consecutive series of 355 patients with increased esophageal exposure to gastric juice is shown in Fig. 1-8.

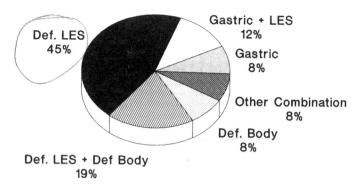

Fig. 1-8   Distribution of the causes of gastroesophageal reflux in a consecutive series of 355 patients with increased esophageal exposure to gastric juice. Def. = defective; LES = lower esophageal sphincter.

Failure of the lower esophageal sphincter can be caused by inadequate pressure, overall length, or intra-abdominal length, the portion of the sphincter exposed to the positive pressure environment of the abdomen. Failure of one or two of the components of the sphincter may be compensated for by the clearance of the esophageal body. Failure of all three sphincter components inevitably leads to increased esophageal exposure to gastric juice. The most common cause of a mechanically defective lower esophageal sphincter is inadequate sphincter pressure most likely caused by an abnormality of myogenic function (Fig. 1-8). A normal sphincter pressure can be nullified by an inadequate abdominal length or by an abnormally short overall length of the sphincter. An adequate abdominal length of sphincter is important in preventing reflux caused by increases in intra-abdominal pressure. An adequate overall length is important to increase the resistance to reflux caused by increases in intragastric pressure independent of intra-abdominal pressure.[14]

The combined effects of sphincter pressure, overall length, and abdominal length can be determined by integrating the radial pressures exerted over the entire length of the sphincter. This can be done by calculating the volume of the three-dimensional sphincter pressure profile, the sphincter pressure vector volume.[15] The three-dimensional sphincter pressure representations of a normal volunteer, a patient with a defective sphincter and Barrett's esophagus, and the same patient after Nissen fundoplication are shown in Fig. 1-9.

A second cause of increased esophageal exposure to gastric juice is inefficient esophageal clearance of refluxed material.[16] This can result in an abnormal esophageal exposure to gastric juice in individuals who have a mechanically intact lower esophageal sphincter and normal gastric function by the failure to clear physiologic reflux. This situation is relatively uncommon, and ineffective clearance is more likely to be seen in association with a mechanically defective sphincter, where it augments the esophageal exposure to gastric juice by prolonging the duration of each reflux episode (Fig. 1-8).

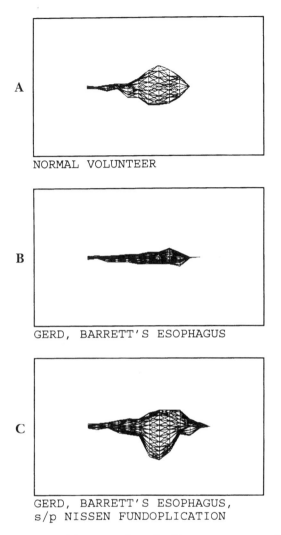

NORMAL VOLUNTEER

GERD, BARRETT'S ESOPHAGUS

GERD, BARRETT'S ESOPHAGUS,
s/p NISSEN FUNDOPLICATION

Fig. 1-9 The three-dimensional lower esophageal sphincter pressure profile in a normal volunteer **(A),** a patient with a mechanically defective sphincter **(B),** and the same patient 1 year following Nissen fundoplication **(C).** (From Stein HJ, DeMeester TR, Naspetti R, et al. The three-dimensional lower esophageal sphincter pressure profile in gastroesophageal reflux disease. Ann Surg 214:374-384, 1991.)

The four factors important in esophageal clearance are gravity, esophageal motor activity, salivation, and anchorage of the distal esophagus in the abdomen. The bulk of refluxed gastric juice is cleared from the esophagus by a primary peristaltic wave initiated by a pharyngeal swallow.[16] Secondary peristalsis initiated by either distention of the lower esophagus or a drop in the intraesophageal pH is less important. Combined video/cine radiographic and manometric studies have shown that failure of esophageal clearance can be detected by nonperistaltic esophageal

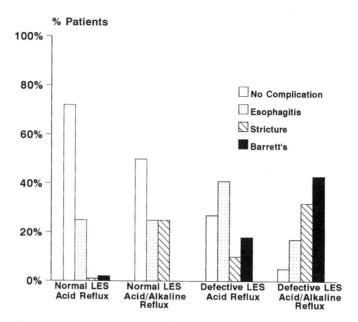

Fig. 1-10   Prevalence and severity of esophageal mucosal injury in patients with only acid reflux and acid/alkaline reflux with or without a mechanically defective lower esophageal sphincter *(LES)*. (From Stein HJ, Barlow AP, DeMeester TR, et al. Complications of gastroesophageal reflux disease: Role of the lower esophageal sphincter, esophageal acid/alkaline exposure, and duodenogastric reflux. Ann Surg 216:35-43, 1992.)

contractions or contractions with low amplitude. Salivation contributes to esophageal clearance by neutralizing the minute amount of acid that is left following a peristaltic wave. The presence of a hiatal hernia can also cause a reduction in the efficiency of acid clearance.

Gastric abnormalities that increase esophageal exposure to gastric juice include gastric dilation, increased intragastric pressure, a persistent gastric reservoir, and increased gastric acid secretion. The effect of gastric dilation is to shorten the overall length of the lower esophageal sphincter resulting in a decrease in the sphincter resistance to reflux. Increased intragastric pressures occur in patients with outlet obstruction due to a scarred pylorus or duodenum, or after vagotomy. The persistence of the gastric reservoir results from delayed gastric emptying secondary to myogenic abnormalities such as is seen in patients with advanced diabetes, diffuse neuromuscular disorders, and post-viral infections. Gastric hypersecretion can increase esophageal exposure to gastric juice by the physiologic reflux of large amounts of concentrated acid.

Complications of gastroesophageal reflux result from the damage inflicted by gastric juice on the esophageal mucosa or the respiratory epithelium and the changes caused by their subsequent repair and fibrosis. Complications of GERD are classified as esophagitis, stricture, and Barrett's esophagus, with its known malignant potential. The presence of the complications of GERD is directly related to the prevalence of a mechanically defective sphincter[17] (Fig. 1-10). This indicates that a mechanically defective sphincter is the major factor in the development of complications of the disease. The observation that a mechanically defective sphincter also occurs in a significant number of patients who do not have a complication of increased esophageal exposure to gastric juice suggests that the defect in the sphincter is primary and not the result of inflammation or tissue damage.

Complications of GERD can also occur in patients with a normal lower esophageal sphincter, while some patients with a defective sphincter do not develop complications. This suggests that the composition of refluxed gastric juice may also be an important factor in the pathogenesis of esophageal mucosal injury. Experimental studies have shown that gastric acid and alkaline duodenogastric reflux interrelate and modulate the content and injurious effects of refluxed gastric juice in the distal esophagus.[18] Clinical studies have confirmed this concept and have shown that patients with increased esophageal exposure to gastric juice, contaminated with alkaline duodenal contents, have a higher prevalence and severity of complications compared to those who have increased esophageal acid exposure only[17] (Fig. 1-10). Complications of GERD are particularly frequent and severe in patients with a mechanically defective sphincter and an alkaline component to the refluxate. These studies suggest that the lower esophageal sphincter is the primary barrier against reflux of any gastric contents and that reflux of gastric juice contaminated with duodenal contents is more detrimental to the esophageal mucosa than reflux of only acid gastric juice.

Secondary Esophageal Motor Disorders

Esophageal motility disorders may also result from more generalized neural, muscular, or metabolic systemic abnormality disturbances or inflammation and neoplasia of the esophagus. The esophagus is particularly affected by almost any of the collagen vascular disorders. The most common are progressive systemic sclerosis, mixed connective tissue disease, polymyositis, and dermatomyositis.[19-21]

Eighty percent of patients with progressive systemic sclerosis have an esophageal motor abnormality. In most cases the disease follows a prolonged course and usually only affects the smooth muscle in the distal two thirds of the esophagus. Typical findings on esophageal manometry are normal peristalsis in the proximal striated esophagus, with weak or absent peristalsis in the distal smooth muscle portion. The lower esophageal sphincter pressure is progressively weakened as the disease advances, resulting in increased esophageal exposure to gastric juice due to a mechanically defective lower esophageal sphincter and poor clearance function of the esophageal body.

In patients with polymyositis or dermatomyositis the upper striated muscle portion is the major site of esophageal involvement causing aspiration, nasopharyngeal regurgitation, and cervical dysphagia. Mixed connective tissue disease shows a mixture of the manometric findings of progressive systemic sclerosis and polymyositis.

REFERENCES

1. Waters PF, DeMeester TR. Foregut motor disorders and their surgical management. Med Clin North Am 65:1237-1272, 1981.
2. Stein HJ, DeMeester TR, Hinder RA. Outpatient physiologic testing and surgical management of foregut motility disorders. Curr Probl Surg 29:415-555, 1992.
3. Friedland GW. Historical review of the changing concepts of lower esophageal anatomy: 430 B.C.-1977. AJR 131:373-388, 1978.
4. Liebermann-Meffert D, Allgower M, Schmid P, et al. Muscular equivalent of the esophageal sphincter. Gastroenterology 76:31-38, 1979.
5. Stein HJ, Liebermann-Meffert D, DeMeester TR, et al. Three-dimensional pressure image and muscular structure of the human lower esophageal sphincter. Surgery 1995 (in press).
6. Cook IJ, Gibb M, Panagopoulos V, et al. Pharyngeal (Zenker's) diverticulum is a disorder of upper esophageal opening. Gastroenterology 103:1229-1235, 1992.
7. Bonavina L, Khan NA, DeMeester TR. Pharyngoesophageal dysfunctions: The role of cricopharyngeal myotomy. Arch Surg 120:541-549, 1985.
8. Vantrappen G, Janssens J, Hellemans J, et al. Achalasia, diffuse esophageal spasm, and related motility disorders. Gastroenterology 76:450-457, 1979.
9. Castell DO, Richter JE, Dalton CB, eds. Esophageal Motility Testing. New York: Elsevier, 1987.
10. Stein HJ, DeMeester TR. Indications, technique, and clinical use of ambulatory 24-hour esophageal motility monitoring in a surgical practice. Ann Surg 217:128-137, 1993.
11. Kahrilas PJ, Dodds WJ, Hogan WJ. Effect of peristaltic dysfunction on esophageal volume clearance. Gastroenterology 94:73-80, 1988.
12. Stein HJ. Ambulatory 24-hour esophageal motility monitoring in patients with primary esophageal motor disorders and/or nonobstructive dysphagia. Dysphagia 8:105-111, 1993.
13. Stein HJ, DeMeester TR, Eypasch EP, et al. Ambulatory 24-hour esophageal manometry in the evaluation of esophageal motor disorders and noncardiac chest pain. Surgery 110:753-763, 1991.
14. Zaninotto G, DeMeester TR, Schwizer W, et al. The lower esophageal sphincter in health and disease. Am J Surg 155:104-111, 1988.
15. Stein HJ, DeMeester TR, Naspetti R, et al. The three-dimensional lower esophageal sphincter pressure profile in gastroesophageal reflux disease. Ann Surg 214:374-384, 1991.
16. Helm JF, Riedel DR, Dodds WJ, et al. Determinants of esophageal acid clearance in normal subjects. Gastroenterology 85:607-612, 1983.
17. Stein HJ, Barlow AP, DeMeester TR, et al. Complications of gastroesophageal reflux disease: Role of the lower esophageal sphincter, esophageal acid/alkaline exposure, and duodenogastric reflux. Ann Surg 216:35-43, 1992.
18. Johnson LF, Harmon JW. Experimental esophagitis in a rabbit model. J Clin Gastroenterol 8 (Suppl):26-44, 1986.
19. Steven MB, Hookman P, Siegel CI, et al. Aperistalsis of the esophagus in patients with connective-tissue disorders and Raynaud's phenomenon. N Engl J Med 270:1218-1222, 1964.
20. Zamhost BJ, Hirschberg J, Ippoliti AF, et al. Esophagitis in scleroderma: Prevalence and risk factors. Gastroenterology 92:421-428, 1987.
21. Marshall JB, Kretschmar JM, Gerhardt DC, et al. Gastrointestinal manifestations of mixed connective tissue disease. Gastroenterology 98:1232-1238, 1990.

2

Preoperative Assessment of Esophageal Function

Mario Costantini, M.D. • *Tom R. DeMeester, M.D.*

The surgical treatment of benign esophageal disease is one of the most challenging fields in surgery in that it alters or reconstructs anatomy with the purpose of improving function. The outcome of surgery is assessed by the ability of the procedure to provide a complete and permanent relief of all symptoms and complications. The recent introduction and widespread use of laparoscopic and thoracoscopic techniques have given a new dimension to esophageal functional surgery. These new approaches have changed the attitude of both patients and physicians toward surgical treatment of esophageal functional disease, but have increased the risk of superficial or improper selection of patients. Symptoms of esophageal disease, such as dysphagia, heartburn, regurgitation, belching, and epigastric and retrosternal pain, are often nonspecific and occur in a variety of esophageal as well as gastric and duodenal disorders.[1] Atypical symptoms of esophageal disease, such as wheezing, choking, coughing, and chest pain, can also mimic other organ abnormalities.[2] Further, anatomic and histologic alterations occur at a late stage and represent end-stage or complications of the functional disease. Consequently, a precise diagnosis must be made prior to any surgical therapy since its purpose is to improve the lasting performance of a malfunctioning organ. A successful result depends on (1) the documentation of esophageal disease as the cause of the patient's symptoms, (2) the understanding of the underlying cause of esophageal dysfunction, and (3) the identification of patients who should have surgical treatment. The surgeon therefore must be sure to perform the right operation for the right disease in the right patient.

A careful preoperative evaluation of a patient with suspected esophageal functional disease should begin by investigating the anatomic alterations and complications of the disease by means of radiology and endoscopy. The objective diagnosis and accurate understanding of the pathophysiologic mechanism of the patient's abnormality can only be assessed by the use of esophageal function tests[3] (Table 2-1). Stationary esophageal manometry, 24-hour pH monitoring of the distal esophagus, and ambulatory 24-hour motility monitoring of the esophageal body are the tests most widely used. New emerging technologies for the detection of duodenogas-

Table 2-1   Tests for the preoperative evaluation of esophageal function*

Tests for the evaluation of esophageal motor function and clearance

Esophageal manometry (body evaluation)
24-hour motility monitoring
Esophageal scintigraphy
Conventional radiology (solid and wet boluses)
Acid clearing test (ACT)

Tests for the evaluation of LES competency

Esophageal manometry (evaluation of the LES)
Standard acid reflux test (SART)
Conventional radiology

Tests for the detection of abnormal exposure of the distal esophagus to gastric and duodenal juice

24-hour pH monitoring
24-hour monitoring of bilirubin

Tests based on the relationship between symptoms and esophageal dysfunction

Pharmacologic provocative test (bethanechol, edrophonium)
Balloon distention test
Acid perfusion test (Bernstein test)
24-hour pH monitoring
24-hour motility monitoring

Tests for the evaluation of complications of esophageal function disease

Conventional radiology
Endoscopy (plus biopsy)

Tests for the evaluation of gastroduodenal function

24-hour pH monitoring of the stomach
Gastric acid analysis
Gastroduodenal manometry
Gastric emptying study
Cholescintigraphy

*Modified from DeMeester TR, Costantini M. Esophageal function tests. In Pearson FG, ed. Esophageal Surgery. New York: Churchill Livingstone, 1995 (in press).

troesophageal reflux are promising. Because esophageal function is closely related to foregut function, there is, on occasion, a need to evaluate gastroduodenal function. There is only a rare indication for esophageal provocative tests.

RADIOLOGY

The radiologic study of the esophagus remains fundamental to the comprehensive evaluation of a patient with esophageal symptoms. It has also gained increasing attention as a functional study when performed concurrently with esopha-

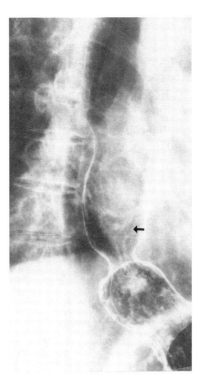

Fig. 2-1   Double contrast x-ray film of the esophagus in a patient with columnar-lined (Barrett's) esophagus. The columnar-lined esophagus reaches the level of the aortic arch and an ulceration is evident in the distal esophagus (arrow).

geal manometry and may give precise information on bolus propagation mechanisms in health and disease.[4,5]

Double-contrast films, obtained by coating the esophagus with dense barium suspension and distending the gullet with gas, provide the best evaluation of the esophageal mucosal surface for the detection of esophagitis or small tumors[6] (Fig. 2-1). Initially, the examination is performed in the prone position to exclude the effect of gravity on bolus propagation. Esophageal motility is assessed by observing multiple (at least five) single swallows of barium. Macroscopic esophageal alterations (hiatal hernias, rings, or strictures) are demonstrated with this technique. The use of solid boluses, such as marshmallow, can be useful in detecting esophageal narrowing, particularly if the examination with fluid barium is unrevealing.[7] A further improvement to the radiographic examination is fluoroscopic observation. Videotape recording of barium swallows (video fluorography) allows repetitive analysis with slow-motion and frame-by-frame playback. This method is particularly useful in evaluating functional disorders of the esophagus and oropharynx. Because of the rapidity and complexity of motor events in the first phases of swallowing, video fluorography is the test of choice for oropharyngeal evaluation.[8,9]

Radiologic evaluation of esophageal function implies the examination of the esophageal body and both sphincters. With swallowing, the relaxation of the upper esophageal sphincter (UES) corresponds to a wide opening of the pharyngoesophageal segment. An abnormal relaxation is seen as a persistent posterior impression from the cricopharyngeal muscle.[8] There is frequently stasis of barium in the piriform sinuses or aspiration. When the barium bolus enters the esophagus, a normal primary peristaltic sequence (or "wave") can be seen as an aboral contraction of the esophageal walls that obliterates the lumen at the top of the barium column and progressively strips the bolus from the esophagus. This corresponds to the onset of

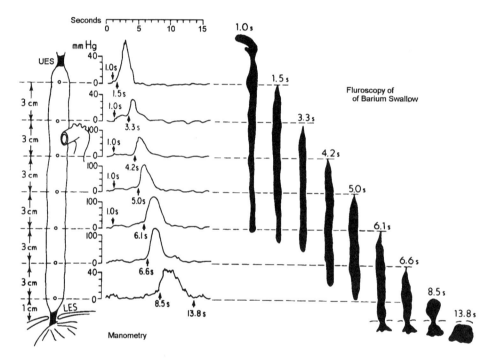

Fig. 2-2 Concurrent manometric and video recording of a 5 ml barium swallow. The tracings from the video images of the fluoroscopic sequence on the right show the distribution of the barium column at the times indicated above the individual tracings and by arrows on the manometric record. In this example, a single peristaltic sequence completely cleared the barium bolus from the esophagus. Pharyngeal injection of barium into the esophagus occurred at the 1.0 second mark. The entry of barium caused distention and a slightly increased intraluminal pressure, indicated by the downward-pointing arrows marked 1.0 second. Shortly thereafter, esophageal peristalsis was initiated. During esophageal peristalsis, luminal closure and the tail of the barium bolus passed each recording site, concurrent with the onset of the manometric pressure wave. Hence, at 1.5 seconds, the peristaltic contraction had just reached the proximal recording site and barium had been stripped from the esophagus proximal to that point. Similarly, at 4.2 seconds, the peristaltic contraction was beginning the third recording site and, correspondingly, the tail of the barium bolus was located at the third recording site. Finally, after completion of the peristaltic contraction (time, 13.8 seconds), all of the barium had been cleared into the stomach. (From Kahrilas PJ, Dodds WJ, Hogan WJ. Effect of peristaltic dysfunction of esophageal volume clearance. Gastroenterology 94:73-80, 1988.)

the peristaltic contraction recorded at manometry[5] (Fig. 2-2). Normally, the peristaltic contraction wave clears all of the barium from the gullet, but occasionally some proximal escape occurs, especially at the level of the aortic arch, where there is the transition from striated to smooth muscle fibers and esophageal contractions are weaker.[4] Abnormal relaxation of the lower esophageal sphincter (LES) is seen as a failure of the esophagogastric junction to distend normally when the bolus arrives, with stasis of barium in the esophageal body.

Radiology should be the first diagnostic test in a patient suffering from dysphagia. It can contribute to the diagnosis with typical findings or, more often, by excluding of organic disease such as neoplasm. In achalasia, a mildly to markedly dilated esophagus is usually detected, with absence of primary peristalsis and a typical beak-like or pencil-like tapering of the esophagogastric junction (Fig. 2-3). The latter represents dysfunction of the LES with a failure of the bolus to distend the tonically contracted sphincter. In the upright position, when the hydrostatic pressure of the barium column in the dilated esophagus overcomes the resting tone of the LES, there is a sudden passage of the barium into the stomach. Another typical finding, present in 50% of patients, is the absence of a gastric air bubble, which represents the inability of normally swallowed air to pass through the contracted sphincter.[10] Particular care must be taken in differentiating true achalasia from so-called "pseudoachalasia" (Fig. 2-4), which is usually caused by neoplastic involvement of the esophagogastric junction or a peptic stricture at this level.

In diffuse esophageal spasm (DES), there may be disruption of peristalsis and nonperistaltic contractions, which often are repetitive and simultaneous and can, in the most advanced cases, cause the typical "corkscrew" appearance of the esophagus (Fig. 2-5). In most cases the radiographic findings in DES may be minimal or nonspecific and the diagnosis must emerge from their correlation with symptoms and the results of esophageal manometry. The same applies to other primary esophageal disorders, such as nutcracker esophagus, hypertensive LES, or nonspecific esophageal motility disorders (NEMDs), as well as to secondary motility disorders, in which radiologic examination can be absolutely normal or can give very nonspecific findings, such as disruption of primary peristalsis with abnormal bolus clearance.[11]

The role of radiologic studies in gastroesophageal reflux disease (GERD) is mostly to detect anatomic complications of the disease, such as ulcerative esophagitis and stricture, although the former is better evaluated with endoscopy. The sensitivity of radiology in detecting gastroesophageal reflux is negligible (34% in a recent review[12]). However, the radiologic examination provides a good estimate of esophageal volume clearance and may demonstrate a need for several swallows to completely empty the esophagus.[11] From the surgical point of view, radiology is important to objectively illustrate the anatomic situation of the esophagogastric junction, the presence and the dimension of a hiatal hernia, and the presence of a shortened esophagus. In this latter case, if antireflux surgery is planned, radiology may suggest a transthoracic approach or a lengthening procedure of the esophagus (Collis gastroplasty).

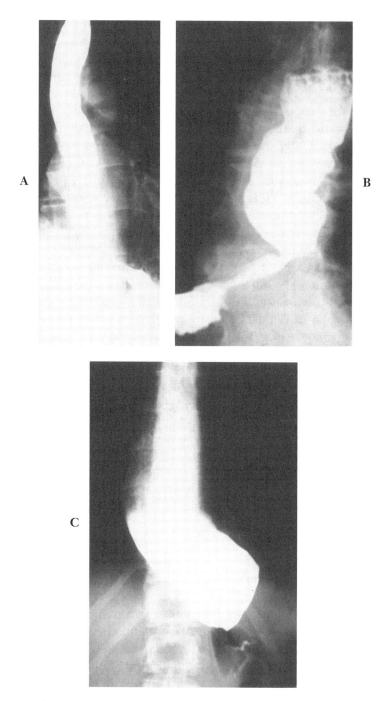

Fig. 2-3   A, Achalasia with mild esophageal dilation and beak-like tapering at lower end of the esophagus, reflecting LES dysfunction. **B,** Achalasia with moderate dilation of the esophagus and some tertiary (spontaneous simultaneous) contractions. **C,** Severe esophageal dilation with sigmoid-shaped esophagus.

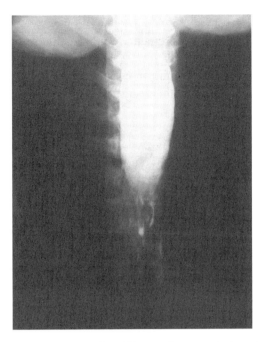

Fig. 2-4 Esophageal dilation and aperistalsis. The esophagogastric junction is irregularly tapered, indicative of a carcinoma of the cardia (pseudoachalasia).

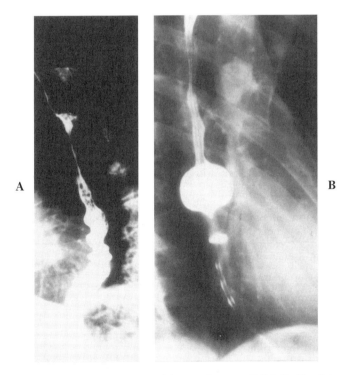

Fig. 2-5 **A,** Typical "corkscrew" appearance of the esophagus in DES. **B,** Simultaneous contractions and pseudodiverticular dilation of the esophageal lumen in a patient with DES.

ENDOSCOPY

Esophagoscopy has become an essential tool in the investigation and diagnosis of upper gastrointestinal disorders. However, it has been estimated that 25% of upper gastrointestinal endoscopies might be unrewarding procedures.[13] The main role of endoscopy in a patient with foregut symptoms is the exclusion of any organic disease, especially malignancy.

In the past, endoscopy was considered the gold standard for the diagnosis of GERD and the presence of esophagitis was diagnostic. With the introduction of 24-hour esophageal pH monitoring techniques, a better definition of GERD based on the abnormal exposure of the distal esophagus to the refluxed gastric juice was made possible[14] and it became evident that only approximately two thirds of patients with GERD had esophagitis at endoscopy.[15] Therefore, endoscopy is not a sensitive method for the diagnosis of GERD (68% sensitivity rate), although it is specific (96%).[16] There are several classifications currently used to score endoscopic esophagitis. The main difference between these systems is in the definition of grade I disease. Some authors accept erythema, uneven color, fuzzy mucosal junction, and friability as the criteria for grade I disease, whereas others do not. Inclusion of these criteria is subject to considerable interobserver variation. Their inclusion increases the sensitivity of endoscopy in detecting mild esophagitis (95%) but compromises the specificity of the test (41%).[16] The Savary-Miller classification system[17] and a simplified endoscopic classification system[15] are summarized in Tables 2-2 and 2-3, respectively.

Histologic examination of biopsy tissue taken during endoscopy may increase the sensitivity of the test in the diagnosis of esophagitis, especially when endoscopic

Table 2-2 The Savary-Miller classification of reflux esophagitis[17]

Grade	Endoscopic Findings
I	One or more supravestibular, nonconfluent mucosal lesions, accompanied by erythema, with or without exudate or superficial erosions
II	Confluent erosive exudative lesions *not* covering the entire circumference
III	Erosive and exudative lesions covering the entire circumference leading to inflammatory infiltration of the wall without stricture
IV	Chronic mucosal lesions (ulcer, fibrosis of wall, stricture, short esophagus, scarring with columnar epithelium)

Table 2-3 Simplified endoscopic classification of esophagitis[15]

Grade	Endoscopic Findings
I	Erythema and friability
II	Linear erosions
III	Deeper and wider erosions with islands of edematous mucosa between erosive furrows
IV	Fibrous stricture or columnar-lined esophagus

appearance of the esophagus is normal. Papillomatosis, basal zone hyperplasia, infiltration of neutrophils and eosinophils, and epithelial erosions and ulcerations are indicative of different severities of esophagitis.[18] However, the accuracy of histology depends on the number of biopsies, their correct orientation and fixation, and the focused interest of the pathologist. Therefore, the usefulness of esophageal histology as an acceptable parameter to judge the severity of GERD has been questioned. Biopsies and brush cytology are necessary for strictures to exclude cancer and to diagnose Barrett's esophagus. Barrett's esophagus is an acquired condition, caused by chronic gastroesophageal reflux, in which the normal squamous mucosa of the distal tubular esophagus is replaced by columnar epithelium (columnar metaplasia). It is the most severe form of reflux esophagitis. Endoscopically, the Z line (or the squamocolumnar junction) appears displaced proximally into the tubular esophagus. In extreme cases this junction can be at the level of the aortic arch or above. In some patients the junction is irregular, with tongues or flame-like extensions of reddish metaplastic mucosa interposed with islands of white squamous epithelium. Histologically, the metaplastic mucosa can be formed by three different types of cells: (1) the gastric fundic type, resembling the mucosa of the fundus of the stomach, with chief and parietal cells; (2) the junctional type, which resembles the gastric cardia epithelium, with cardiac mucous glands but no chief or parietal cells; and (3) the specialized intestinal columnar epithelium, which is found nowhere else in the gastrointestinal tract and has villi and goblet cells.[19] Because of its documented precancerous nature,[20] endoscopic and biopsy surveillance is necessary to detect dysplasia and early malignancies, when cure is still possible. Multiple biopsies and brushings are necessary because high-grade dysplasia and carcinoma can be present without apparent visible abnormality. For accurate mapping, biopsies should be taken circumferentially at every centimeter of the metaplastic mucosa from the esophagogastric junction.

Endoscopy plays little role in the diagnosis of esophageal motility disorders, apart from being useful to exclude neoplastic disease. In the early stage of achalasia, and in other primary and secondary motility disorders, endoscopy can be completely normal. In advanced stages of achalasia, endoscopy reveals a dilated, tortuous esophagus, which is often filled with food, and a whitish, cobblestone-like esophageal mucosa (stasis esophagitis). The gastroesophageal junction is tightly closed and fails to relax with swallowing or distention of the esophagus with air. Negotiation of the endoscope through the LES often requires gentle pressure. The scope has been described as "popping" into the stomach when the sphincter pressure has been overcome. However, the major role of endoscopy is to differentiate true achalasia from pseudoachalasia, which is usually tumor-induced. In this setting, the careful observation of the esophagogastric junction from below, with the scope retroflexed, is mandatory.

STATIONARY ESOPHAGEAL MANOMETRY

Esophageal manometry is the gold standard for assessment of function of the LES and body of the esophagus. It has allowed the identification of primary esophageal motility disorders, such as achalasia, diffuse esophageal spasm, nutcracker esophagus, and hypertensive LES, as well as systemic disorders affecting the esophagus, such as scleroderma, dermatomyositis, mixed connective tissue disease, diabetes, and alcoholic neuropathy. In the preoperative evaluation of GERD, esophageal manometry is necessary to identify a defective LES and deterioration of esophageal body function.

Esophageal manometry is normally performed using low-compliance water-perfused catheters with lateral side holes connected to external transducers. These catheters are made by combining three to eight capillary tubes 0.8 mm in inner diameter with side openings at different levels. Side holes arranged radially at the same level are ideal for measuring pressures circumferentially around the asymmetric LES and UES. Side holes spaced 5 cm apart are necessary for the study of the esophageal peristaltic activity. To obtain maximal information during a single intubation and a minimum number of swallows, most laboratories use an eight-lumen catheter with four side holes at the same level arranged at 90 degrees to each other. The remaining four holes are placed at 5 cm intervals along the length of the catheter. The water infusion is obtained by a low-compliance pneumohydraulic capillary infusion system with a constant infusion rate of 0.6 ml/min.[21]

The study is usually performed after an overnight fast. The catheter is passed through the nose and esophagus into the stomach and the gastric pressure pattern is confirmed. To identify the high-pressure zone of the LES, the catheter is withdrawn across the cardia (Fig. 2-6, *A*). Although some clinicians advocate a steady, rapid withdrawal (rapid pull-through) with the patient holding his or her breath,[22] it has been demonstrated that a stepwise withdrawal of the catheter at 0.5 or 1.0 cm intervals (station pull-through [SPT])[23] provides reproducible and more quantita-

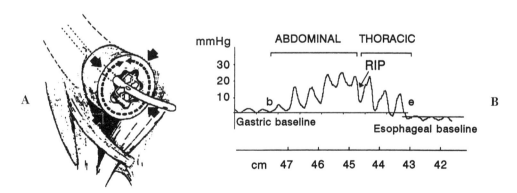

Fig. 2-6   A, Schematic illustration shows measurement of LES pressure with a perfused catheter system. The outflow of the perfusate through the side holes (white arrows) is restricted by the circular muscle tone of the cardia (broken arrow) and the externally applied intra-abdominal pressure (black arrows). **B,** The length of the abdominal and thoracic portion of the LES can be measured on the pressure record by identifying the point where respiratory excursion changes from positive to negative. This is the respiratory inversion point *(RIP)* and is the point where the resting pressure of the LES is measured. b = beginning; e = end of the sphincter.

tive information[24] and allows the patient to breathe normally during the procedure. As the pressure-sensitive station is brought across the gastroesophageal junction, a rise in pressure on the gastric baseline identifies the beginning of the LES (Fig. 2-6, *B*). The respiratory inversion point (RIP) is identified when the positive excursions that occur with breathing in the abdominal cavity change to negative deflections in the thorax. The RIP serves as a reference point at which the amplitude of LES pressure and the length of the sphincter exposed to abdominal pressure are measured. As the pressure-sensitive station is withdrawn into the body of the esophagus, the upper border of the LES is identified by the drop in pressure to the esophageal baseline. From these measurements, the pressure, abdominal length, and overall length of the sphincter are determined (Fig. 2-6, *B*). To account for the asymmetry of the sphincter,[25] the values obtained with the four radial side holes are averaged.

Recently, to improve the SPT technique, a new method, the slow motorized pull-through technique (sMPT) has been introduced to evaluate the LES. It consists of pulling back the catheter at a constant rate (1.0 mm/sec) using a motor. This technique is quick, approximately 1 minute for a passage through the sphincter, and well accepted by the patient. It allows high-fidelity tracings without swallowing artifacts, even in most difficult patients (Fig. 2-7). Since the pull-through is performed in a continuous mode, it provides an accurate determination of sphincter length, without the approximation (± 0.5 to 1.0 cm) given by the SPT technique. Because the patient is allowed to breathe normally, it is possible to locate the RIP, from which the abdominal length can be calculated. Since the technique is inde-

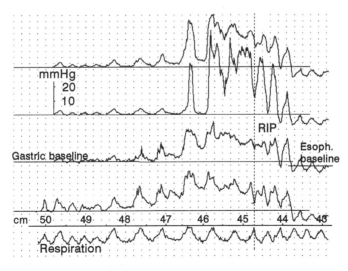

Fig. 2-7 Manometric tracing of a LES pressure obtained with four side holes located at the same level and positioned radially at 90 degrees to each other. The sMPT technique was used. The asymmetry of the sphincter is evident. The sphincter is longer in the lower tracing and the pressure is higher in the upper tracing. (From DeMeester TR, Constantini M. Esophageal function tests. In Pearson FG, ed. Esophageal Surgery. New York: Churchill Livingstone, 1995 [in press].)

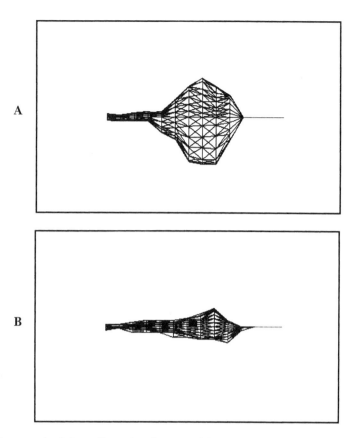

Fig. 2-8 Computerized three-dimensional image of the LES in a healthy volunteer **(A)** and in a patient with Barrett's esophagus **(B).** A catheter with four to eight radial side holes is withdrawn through the gastroesophageal junction. The radially measured pressures are plotted around an axis representing gastric baseline pressure. The volume inscribed by the three-dimensional image (sphincter vector volume) can be calculated, giving the best estimate of the LES mechanical effectiveness in the prevention of reflux of gastric juice from the stomach into the esophagus.

pendent of the operator, it lends itself to automated computer analysis. Comparison of the technique with the traditional SPT technique in a group of healthy volunteers and patients with different esophageal disorders revealed a good correlation for pressure, overall length, and abdominal length.[26] Further, by using the four radially oriented side holes positioned at the same level, a three-dimensional pressure image of the sphincter can be constructed by plotting the pressure values radially around an axis representing the gastric baseline[27] (Fig. 2-8). The volume circumscribed by the three-dimensional sphincter image, the so-called "vector volume"[28] integrates pressures exerted over the entire length and around the circumference of the sphincter into one number, representing sphincter resistance to reflux of gastric contents. This measure can be calculated using standard trigonometric formulas and is expressed in units of mm $Hg^2 \times$ mm. Using the SPT or the sMPT techniques, the RIP can be identified, and the intrathoracic and intra-

Table 2-4   Normal lower esophageal sphincter parameters in 50 healthy volunteers

	Mean	SEM	Median	Percentiles	
				5th	95th
Pressure (mm Hg)	13.8	0.7	13.0	8.0	26.5
Overall length (cm)	3.7	0.2	3.6	2.6	5.4
Abdominal length (cm)	2.2	0.2	2.0	1.1	3.4
Intra-abdominal SVV (mm Hg^2 × mm)	3613	531	2012	684	12918
Total SVV (mm Hg^2 × mm)	5723	843	3667	1212	16780

SEM = standard error of the mean; SVV = sphincter vector volume.

abdominal portions of the volume, the portions of sphincter pressure vector volume located above and below the RIP, can be calculated separately. Table 2-4 shows the values of LES pressure, overall length, length of the abdominal segment, and sphincter vector volume in 50 asymptomatic subjects, with the range of normality (5th to 95th percentiles).

For the evaluation of sphincter relaxation and postrelaxation characteristics, the side holes located 5 cm apart are used. One side hole is repositioned within the high pressure zone, a distal one is located in the stomach, and a proximal one is positioned within the esophageal body. Five to 10 wet swallows (5 ml water) are performed. In the normal situation the sphincter pressure should drop to the level of gastric pressure during each wet swallow.

The function of the esophageal body is assessed with the five recording sites located at various levels in the esophagus. To standardize the procedure, the most proximal pressure transducer is located 1 cm below the well-defined cricopharyngeal sphincter, with the distal orifices trailing at 5 cm intervals over the whole length of the esophagus. Using this method, a pressure response throughout the whole esophagus can be obtained on swallowing (Fig. 2-9). The response to 10 wet swallows is recorded. Dry swallows were less reliable and therefore were generally abandoned.[29] Amplitude, duration, and morphology, that is, the number of peaks and repetitive activity of contractions following each swallow, are calculated at all recorded levels of the esophageal body. The delay between the onset or peak of esophageal contractions at the various levels in the esophagus is used to calculate the speed of wave propagation. The esophageal contraction waves following a swallow are classified as peristaltic, simultaneous, interrupted, or dropped (Fig. 2-10). Modern computer technology allows an objective and quick analysis of these parameters. Manometric values at the different esophageal levels obtained in a group of 136 healthy subjects with a wide range of age are shown in Table 2-5 and form the reference values used in our laboratory.[30]

Based on simultaneous manometry and video fluorography, Kahrilas, Dodds, and Hogan[5] showed that an adequate amplitude of contraction and propagation speeds was required to clear the esophagus of a bolus of liquid barium in the supine position. They classified contraction sequences as effective, possibly effective, or in-

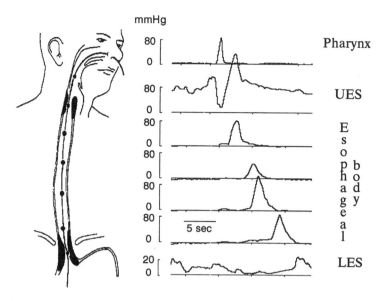

Fig. 2-9 Schematic representation of normal esophageal peristalsis initiated by a pharyngeal swallow and coordinated with relaxation of the upper and lower esophageal sphincters.

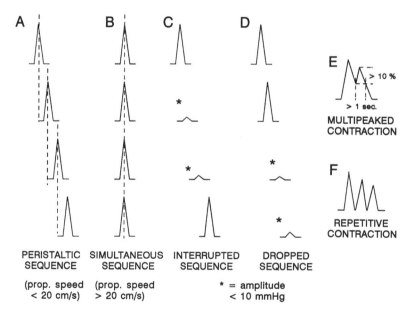

Fig. 2-10 Graphic representation of the classification of esophageal contraction waves on stationary manometry. A complete peristaltic sequence **(A)** is a series of detectable contractions at each esophageal level, with a progression speed slower than 20 cm/sec (i.e., the time between the peak axes of two adjacent contractions). Simultaneous sequence **(B)** is a series of detectable contractions at each esophageal level, with a progression speed faster than 20 cm/sec. An interrupted sequence **(C)** is a series of detectable contractions in which an initial contraction is followed by no detectable contractions (<10 mm Hg), with a normal contraction subsequently reappearing. The dropped sequence **(D)** is a series of detectable contractions in which an initial contraction is followed by *no* detectable contractions (<10 mm Hg). The morphology of the contractions is classified as normal, multipeaked, or repetitive. The difference between multipeaked **(E)** and repetitive **(F)** contractions is that the pressure between two consecutive peaks returns to the baseline in the latter. (From DeMeester TR, Costantini M. Esophageal function tests. In Pearson FG, ed. Esophageal Surgery. New York: Churchill Livingstone, 1995 [in press].)

Table 2-5 Median values and range of normality (5th to 95th percentiles) for manometric parameters of esophageal body obtained by wet and dry swallows in 136 normal subjects

	Level	Wet Swallows	Dry Swallows
Amplitude (mm Hg)	I	88 (40-177)	74 (26-154)
	II	40 (14-94)	28 (14-74)
	III	76 (30-164)	52 (26-142)
	IV	93 (38-180)	61 (20-148)
	V	93 (36-190)	78 (22-172)
Duration (sec)	I	2.3 (1.5-4.3)	2.3 (1.5-3.9)
	II	3.1 (1.8-4.8)	2.8 (1.0-4.5)
	III	3.3 (2.4-5.2)	3.1 (1.8-4.6)
	IV	3.6 (2.6-5.7)	3.4 (2.0-5.6)
	V	3.7 (2.4-7.0)	3.6 (2.4-6.4)
Velocity (cm/sec)	I-II	2.4 (1.5-4.6)	2.8 (1.6-6.2)
	II-III	2.8 (1.9-6.2)	3.1 (1.9-8.3)
	III-IV	3.8 (1.9-8.3)	4.5 (1.8-8.3)
	IV-V	2.6 (1.3-8.3)	3.5 (1.7-12.5)
	I-V	2.9 (2.1-4.0)	3.5 (2.2-5.0)
Simultaneous (%)	I-II	0 (0-10)	0 (0-10)
	II-III	0 (0-10)	0 (0-20)
	III-IV	0 (0-10)	0 (0-20)
	IV-V	0 (0-10)	0 (0-40)
Interrupted (%)	I	0 (0-0)	0 (0-10)
	II	0 (0-20)	0 (0-30)
	III	0 (0-10)	0 (0-30)
	IV	0 (0-10)	0 (0-30)
	V	0 (0-10)	0 (0-30)
Dropped (%)	II	0 (0-10)	0 (0-20)
	III	0 (0-10)	0 (0-30)
	IV	0 (0-10)	0 (0-30)

effective. Effective sequences were defined as peristaltic contractions with a minimum amplitude of 18 mm Hg at the first esophageal level, 25 mm Hg at the second level, 30 mm Hg at the third and fourth levels, and 43 mm Hg at the fifth level. Possibly effective sequences were peristaltic with amplitudes higher than 10 mm Hg (first and second levels), 20 mm Hg (third and fourth levels), or 25 mm Hg (fifth esophageal level). Ineffective sequences were those sequences below these thresholds, or which had any interrupted, dropped, or simultaneous contractions.

The position, length, and pressure of the UES are evaluated by a SPT technique, with 0.5 to 1.0 cm increments from the cervical esophagus to the pharynx. To account for the anatomic asymmetry of the UES,[31] the values obtained from the side holes oriented in the different directions must be averaged. The function of the UES on swallowing is evaluated placing one side hole of the catheter in the pharynx, one in the proximal part of the sphincter, and one in the upper esophagus. Because of the short duration of the pharyngeal swallowing phase (1.5 seconds), high-speed graphic recordings (50 mm/sec) are necessary to evaluate the coordination of cricopharyngeal relaxation with hypopharyngeal contraction. Normally, pharyngeal contractions reach 50 to 60 mm Hg and are coordinated with complete UES relaxation (i.e., a fall in the sphincter pressure to the less-than-atmospheric intraesophageal pressure).

Orad mobility of the UES during swallowing (2 to 3 cm) may give a misleading impression of its relaxation since a single side hole, positioned in the center of the UES at rest, may actually lie in the cervical esophagus during a swallow.[32] To obviate this problem, a dedicated special catheter assembly, consisting of eight side holes located at 1.0 cm intervals and oriented radially around the catheter, can be used.[33] Experience has shown this to be useful in evaluating the UES relaxation and the pharyngoesophageal coordination (Fig. 2-11, *A*). An alternative approach is to use a particular type of sleeve sensor,[34] made especially for the evaluation of UES relaxation over long periods of time. This device is a reliable indicator of UES relaxation. Its disadvantages are its slow response rate to pressure rises and its large caliber, both of which must be taken into account in evaluating resting pressure values. Further, because water-perfused catheters, even with a low compliance and good pressure rise rate (>200 mm Hg/sec), may be inadequate to study rapid changes in pharyngeal pressure, which may reach up to 500 mm Hg/sec, some authors advocate the use of solid-state microtransducers.[35]

Stationary esophageal manometry, performed as described above, is indicated

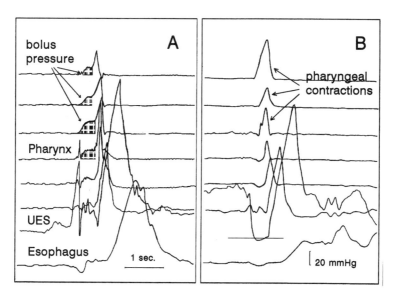

Fig. 2-11   A, Normal cricopharyngeal recording made with a catheter with side holes spaced 1 cm apart. This technique shows the relation of pharyngeal contractions to the relaxation of the UES and response in the cervical esophagus. In this patient with Zenker's diverticulum, a nonrelaxing UES and a prominent intrabolus or "shoulder" pressure before the upstroke of pharyngeal contractions are evident. **B,** Myotomy increased the compliance of the pharyngoesophageal segment, with complete disappearance of the "shoulder" pressure in the pharyngeal contractions. (From DeMeester TR, Costantini M. Esophageal function tests. In Pearson FG, ed. Esophageal Surgery. New York: Churchill Livingstone, 1995 [in press].)

when (1) a motility disorder of the esophageal body and/or the LES is suspected from symptoms of dysphagia, regurgitation, or chest pain; (2) a comprehensive evaluation of the antireflux mechanism in GERD is desired; or (3) a disturbance of the pharyngoesophageal phase of swallowing is suspected.

Functional Disorders of the Esophageal Body and LES

Abnormalities occurring in the worm-drive pump of the esophageal body or the LES give rise to a number of disorders in the esophageal phase of swallowing. These disorders are due to either a direct deterioration of esophageal muscle function (primary motility disorders) or a more generalized neural, muscular, or systemic disease, such as progressive systemic sclerosis, dermatomyositis, or myasthenia gravis (secondary motility disorders). With the introduction of esophageal manometry a number of primary esophageal motility disorders have been classified as separate disease entities, based on amplitude, duration, progression, and nature of the esophageal contractions and on function of the LES on swallowing (Table 2-6).

Table 2-6 Characteristic and diagnostic criteria for primary esophageal motility disorders on standard manometry

Achalasia

Incomplete lower esophageal sphincter relaxation (<75% relaxation)*
Aperistalsis in the esophageal body
Elevated lower esophageal sphincter resting pressure (>26 mm Hg)*
Increased intraesophageal baseline pressures relative to gastric baseline*

Diffuse esophageal spasm

Simultaneous (nonperistaltic contractions)(>20% of wet swallows)
Intermittent normal peristalsis
Repetitive and multipeaked contractions*
Spontaneous contractions*
Contractions of increased amplitude and duration*

Nutcracker esophagus

Mean peristaltic amplitude in the distal esophagus >180 mm Hg
Normal peristaltic sequence
Mean duration of contractions in the distal esophagus >7 seconds*

Hypertensive lower esophageal sphincter

Elevated lower esophageal sphincter resting pressure (>26 mm Hg)
Normal lower esophageal sphincter relaxation
Normal peristalsis in the esophageal body

Nonspecific esophageal motility disorders

Decreased or absent amplitude of esophageal peristalsis
Increased number of nontransmitted contractions
Abnormal waveforms
Normal mean lower esophageal sphincter pressure and relaxation

*Frequent finding, but not required for the diagnosis.

These specific primary disorders are achalasia, diffuse or segmental esophageal spasm, high-amplitude peristaltic esophageal contractions, the so-called "nutcracker esophagus," and the hypertensive LES. The term "nonspecific esophageal motor disorder" (NEMD) includes patients whose manometric features are clearly abnormal but defy classification into one of the major groups. The pathogenesis, clinical aspects, and treatment of these conditions are beyond the scope of this chapter. Fig. 2-12 illustrates the typical findings in achalasia, DES, and nutcracker

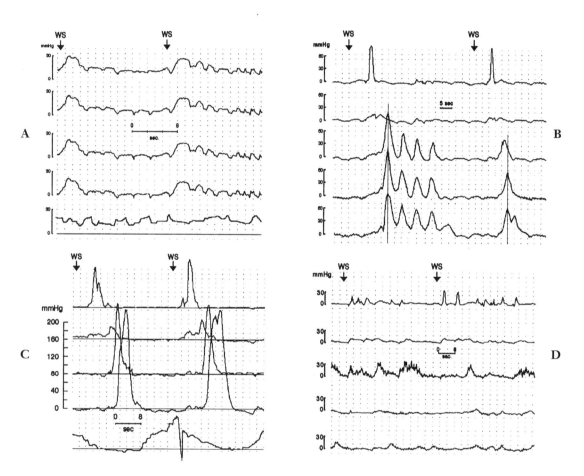

Fig. 2-12 **A,** Esophageal motility in a patient with achalasia, showing the typical features: absence of peristaltic progression in the esophageal body and the inability of the LES to completely relax on swallowing. **B,** Esophageal body motility in a patient with DES. The motor disorder is characterized by an increased percentage of simultaneous contractions (>20%). The contractions can be repetitive, multipeaked, with high amplitude and long duration. The second level from the top is at the junction of striated and smooth muscle where contractions are normally of low amplitude. **C,** Esophageal motility in a patient with nutcracker esophagus. Esophageal contractions are always peristaltic, with high amplitude (>180 mm Hg). LES relaxation is maintained. **D,** Esophageal motility in a patient with progressive systemic sclerosis. A weak motor activity is maintained in the upper esophagus, whereas in the distal two thirds (smooth muscle) there is a virtual absence of any detectable activity in response to swallow. WS = wet swallow.

esophagus. A careful identification of these disorders is crucial because there are reports of devastating results of an erroneous treatment for a mistaken esophageal motor disorder.[36]

Although the most common disease leading to secondary deterioration of esophageal body function is long-standing GERD, the term usually denotes an esophageal motility disorder resulting from a generalized neural, muscular, or systemic metabolic disturbance. In these cases, manometric findings are often nonspecific, resembling those observed in NEMD. The only exception is progressive systemic sclerosis, in which the typical findings are normal peristalsis in the proximal striated esophagus, with weak or absent peristalsis in the distal smooth muscle portion (Fig. 2-12, *D*). The LES pressure is progressively weakened as the disease advances, resulting in increased esophageal exposure to gastric juice due to a mechanically defective LES and poor clearance function of the esophageal body.[37] Identification of this condition is particularly important because aggressive antireflux treatment is required.

Gastroesophageal Reflux Disease

GERD is a common foregut disorder, complicated by esophagitis, stricture, or Barrett's esophagus in approximately two thirds of affected patients.[15] The basic pathophysiologic abnormality in this condition is an increased esophageal exposure to gastric juice. A mechanically defective LES accounts for approximately 60% of GERD.[38] The identification of this cause is important because medical therapy in this situation is plagued by high failure and relapse rates.[39,40] In a group of patients affected with pH-proved GERD, 43% of patients with a normal LES were able to discontinue medical therapy. In the group of patients with a defective LES, medical therapy was also effective, but symptoms recurred whenever therapy was discontinued. On the other hand, 95% of patients with a defective LES who underwent a Nissen antireflux procedure were free of symptoms[40] (Fig. 2-13).

Incompetence of the LES is caused by inadequate pressure, overall length, or abdominal length (i.e., the portion exposed to the positive pressure environment of the abdomen measured on manometry).[38] The probability of increased exposure to gastric juice is 69% to 76% if one component of the sphincter is abnormal, 65% to 88% if two components are abnormal, and 92% if all three components are abnormal. This indicates that the failure of one or two of the components of the sphincter may be compensated for by the clearance of the esophageal body. Failure of all three sphincter components inevitably leads to increased esophageal exposure to gastric juice.

The overall competency of the LES is currently best represented by the calculation of the sphincter vector volume, which combines pressures exerted over the entire length of the sphincter. When measured in a large number of patients, both the total and abdominal sphincter vector volumes were found to be markedly lower in patients with increased esophageal acid exposure compared with healthy volunteers, and the volume decreased with increased severity of mucosal injury.[27] Comparison of sphincter vector volume with standard sphincter parameters (i.e., resting

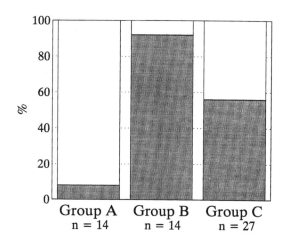

Fig. 2-13 Graph representing the need for continuous medications in patients affected by pH-proved GERD and followed up for a period of 6 to 60 months. Group A were patients with a defective LES who underwent surgery (Nissen fundoplication). Group B were patients with a defective LES who refused surgery and preferred medical treatment. Group C were patients with a normal LES who underwent medical treatment. In group C, 44% of the patients were able to discontinue the treatment and were free of symptoms. In group B, symptoms recurred in all but one patient when therapy was discontinued (unpublished data).

pressure, overall length, and abdominal length) showed that sphincter vector volume had no significant advantage in detecting a defective sphincter in patients with severe GERD and advanced complications. Sphincter vector volume did have a greater sensitivity than standard manometry in identifying a mechanically defective sphincter in patients with increased esophageal acid exposure but no mucosal damage.[27] In a different series of patients, calculation of sphincter vector volume confirmed an increased accuracy of esophageal manometry in detecting a defective LES.[41] Therefore, computer-aided manometry with the calculation of the sphincter pressure vector volume should become the standard technique to assess sphincter competence.

A second cause of increased esophageal exposure to gastric juice is inefficient esophageal clearance of refluxed material.[42] This can result in an abnormal esophageal exposure to gastric juice in individuals who have a mechanically normal LES and normal gastric function by ineffectual clearing of physiologic reflux episodes. This situation is relatively uncommon, and ineffectual clearance is more apt to be seen in association with a mechanically incompetent cardia, where it augments the esophageal exposure to gastric juice by prolonging the duration of each reflux episode.

Finally, abnormal body function can affect the choice of surgical antireflux procedure to be performed. Poor motility is associated with an increased prevalence of postoperative dysphagia when a full 360-degree fundoplication is performed. A partial fundoplication should be the procedure of choice in this situation.

Pharyngoesophageal Swallowing Disorders

Disorders of the pharyngoesophageal phase of swallowing are relatively uncommon. They result from a incoordination of the neuromuscular events during the act of swallowing and the inability to propel the swallowed material from the oropharynx into the cervical esophagus. Zenker's diverticulum or cricopharyngeal bar is often, but not always, present.

The rapidity of the oropharyngeal phase of swallowing, the movement of the gullet, and the asymmetry of the cricopharyngeus account for the difficulty in assessing abnormalities of esophagopharyngeal swallowing disorders with manometric techniques. However, carefully performed motility studies may demonstrate incoordination and incomplete relaxation of the UES during swallowing. This pattern is a feature of many neurologic diseases, including cerebrovascular accidents, or trauma, including head injury and iatrogenic nerve injury.[43] It may result in failure of the pharynx to empty and cause dysphagia, nasal regurgitation, and aspiration. In other patients, particularly those with a history of poliomyelitis, the pressure generated by the pharynx may be subnormal, <25 mm Hg, which represents the lower limit of the normal range.[44] This is important to identify because symptoms in the presence of a profound loss of pharyngeal pressure may be alleviated by a cricopharyngeal myotomy.

It has been difficult to consistently demonstrate a motility abnormality in patients with cervical dysphagia, cricopharyngeal bar, or Zenker's diverticulum, suggesting that, if present, their effects are subtle and do not justify a major etiologic role. Recent studies[45,46] focused attention on the role of a reduced compliance of the UES in the pathophysiology of these disorders, making a distinction between a "manometrically relaxed" and "anatomically relaxed" sphincter (Fig. 2-14). Com-

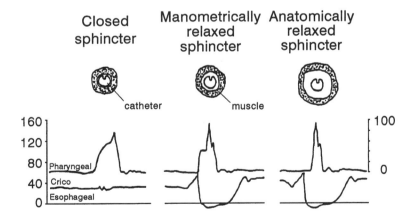

Fig. 2-14 The intrabolus pressure in the hypopharynx, or shoulder pressure, in a manometrically relaxed but incompletely anatomically relaxed UES. The shoulder on the pharyngeal pressure wave indicates resistance to the passage of a bolus through the pharyngoesophageal segment caused by pathology of the cricopharyngeal and cervical esophageal muscle, resulting in poor compliance and incomplete anatomic relaxation. (From Stein HJ, DeMeester TR, Hinder RA. Outpatient physiologic testing and surgical management of foregut motility disorders. Curr Probl Surg 24:418-555, 1992.)

bined radiographic and manometric studies have highlighted the importance of the intrabolus pressure, detected as a "shoulder" or "hump" just before the upstroke of the hypopharyngeal pressure wave, as an indication of a manometrically relaxed but incompletely anatomically relaxed sphincter. It has been shown in two separate studies of patients with Zenker's diverticulum[45] and cricopharyngeal bar[46] that the intrabolus pressure is elevated, despite complete manometric relaxation of the UES. This phenomenon is attributed to decreased compliance of the striated muscle in the cervical esophagus, which allows manometric relaxation but incomplete opening of the sphincter. A higher driving pressure transmitted to the bolus by the tongue and soft palate serves to compensate for the lack of compliance of the upper esophagus. The loss of compliance of the pharyngocervical esophageal segment may be the most common abnormality in patients with pharyngeal dysphagia, with or without Zenker's diverticulum. Increasing the diameter of this noncompliant segment by a surgical myotomy reduces the resistance it imposes to the bolus transport into the esophagus. Manometrically, this results in the disappearing of the "shoulder" in the pharyngeal contraction (see Fig. 2-11, *B*).

AMBULATORY 24-HOUR MOTILITY MONITORING OF THE ESOPHAGUS

The intermittent and unpredictable occurrence of motor abnormalities and symptoms in patients with esophageal motility disorders limits the diagnostic value of standard manometry performed in a laboratory setting over a short time period. The new technique of prolonged esophageal manometry was developed to overcome these shortcomings. Due to the high sampling frequency required to evaluate esophageal motor activity, prolonged outpatient monitoring of esophageal motility became available only after the introduction of portable digital data recorders with a large storage capacity. Data loggers with high storage capacities (4.0 megabytes) allow the evaluation of esophageal motor function based on more than 1000 contraction sequences monitored under a variety of physiologic conditions, that is, upright activity, eating, sleeping, and during symptom periods. Three esophageal pressure channels, one pharyngeal pressure channel, and two pH channels can be used simultaneously for complete foregut physiologic ambulatory monitoring (Fig. 2-15).

The test is performed on an outpatient basis. After the standard stationary manometry, a catheter with four electronic microtransducers is passed through the nose into the esophagus. The three distal transducers, which are 5 cm apart from each other, are positioned 5, 10, and 15 cm above the upper border of the LES. The most proximal transducer, which is 10 cm from the others, is located in the cricopharyngeal area to record pharyngeal swallowing. The transducers are calibrated at 0 and 50 mm Hg by immersion in a water column before and after the test. Eventual drifts must not exceed 8 mm Hg to make the test reliable. The transducers are connected to a portable digital data logger (Microdigitrapper 4.0; Synectics Medical, Dallas, Tex.), and data are stored at an 8 Hz sampling rate. After placement of the catheter, the patients are sent home and encouraged to perform

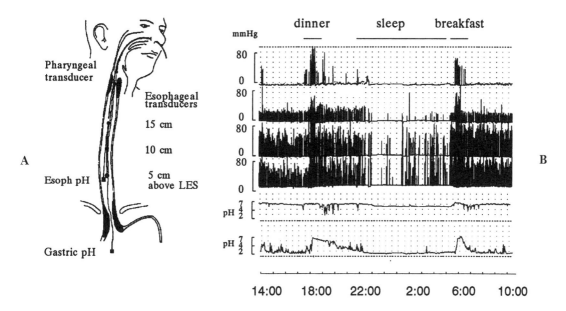

Fig. 2-15 A, Prolonged esophageal motility monitoring is performed with three electronic micro-transducers positioned 5, 10, and 15 cm above the upper border of the LES. An additional micro-transducer is located in the pharynx to detect pharyngeal swallows. Concomitant pH monitoring of the distal esophagus (electrode 5 cm above the LES) and of the stomach (electrode 5 cm below the LES) can be performed. This allows a complete ambulatory foregut physiologic monitoring. **B,** Complete 24-hour foregut ambulatory monitoring in a healthy subject. From top to bottom: compressed pharyngeal swallowing record; compressed esophageal motility record at 15, 10, and 5 cm above the LES; esophageal pH record; and gastric pH record. Increase in swallows and esophageal motility with meals is evident, together with the typical rising in gastric pH (prandial plateau), followed by slow return to the baseline (postprandial decline phase). During sleep, a marked reduction in swallowing and esophageal activity is normal.

normal daily activities. They are instructed to keep a detailed diary for the next 24 hours. The diary should include the time of meals, when they assume the supine position for sleep, when they arise in the morning, and when symptoms occur.

After the test, the raw data are transferred to a computer for further analysis. Approximately 1000 to 1400 contractions are recorded by each pressure transducer over the 24-hour period and a fully automated analysis of such an amount of data is mandatory. A software program for automated computer analysis of 24-hour esophageal motility monitoring (Multigram 6.0; Gastrosoft, Inc., Irving, Tex.) was recently developed and validated against manual analysis.[47] In brief, the esophageal baseline is reset every 60 seconds according to the mode value for that time period. Contraction recognition is based on an algorithm that defines a contraction as a rise in pressure greater than a threshold value for a specified period of time. An amplitude threshold of 15 mm Hg and a duration threshold of 1.0 second showed the best sensitivity and specificity for contraction detection.[47] Most of the artifacts (cough, sneeze, etc.) are usually rejected by these thresholds. Algorithms based on contraction slope and morphology are employed to differentiate artifacts and repetitive contractions. Recognized contractions are then related to each other in esophageal "sequences" or "waves" and classified as peristaltic, simultaneous (if the propagation speed exceeds 20 cm/sec), interrupted (a sequence lacking a contraction in the proximal or middle esophageal channel, but reappearing in the last channel), or dropped (a sequence in which the contractions are present only in the proximal and/or middle channel, but absent in the distal one). The esophageal sequences are also related to pharyngeal swallowing and further classified as primary or secondary. The final report graphically displays amplitude, duration, propagation speed, and characteristics of the detected contractions against a background of

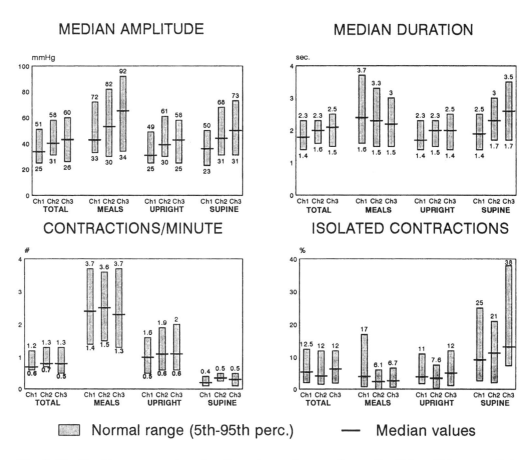

Fig. 2-16 Graphic representation of median values and range of normality (5th to 95th percentiles) for esophageal contractions recorded at different levels during 24-hour ambulatory manometry. During meals there is an increase in the median amplitude and frequency of esophageal contractions. At night the frequency of contractions drops dramatically with an increase in isolated contractions (i.e., unrelated to contractions in other channels). The numbers represent the upper and lower limits of normal. Ch1 = recording site 15 cm above LES; Ch2 = recording site 10 cm above LES; Ch3 = recording site 5 cm above LES. (From DeMeester TR, Costantini M. Esophageal function tests. In Pearson FG, ed. Esophageal Surgery. New York: Churchill Livingstone, 1995 [in press].)

normal for the total period of the test and separately for predefined periods, that is, meal period, upright and supine periods, and periods related to pain or gastro-esophageal reflux. Further, because it has been demonstrated that to clear the esophagus of a liquid bolus, esophageal contractions must be peristaltic and have an adequate amplitude,[5] a classification of sequences into effective (peristaltic contractions and with amplitude above 20, 25, and 30 mm Hg, respectively, at 15, 10, and 5 cm above the LES), possibly effective (peristaltic contractions with amplitude less than these values but higher than 15 mm Hg), and ineffective (simultaneous, interrupted, or dropped contractions) can be obtained for the overall and different periods. This allows a complete quantitative and qualitative evaluation of the patient's esophageal motility during an entire circadian cycle. The median values and the range of normality (5th to 95th percentiles) of some of these parameters obtained in a group of 20 healthy volunteers are represented in Figs. 2-16 to 2-18.

Since its introduction in the middle 1980s, ambulatory esophageal manometry has been primarily used to identify esophageal motility abnormalities as the cause of noncardiac chest pain. Initial experience often showed a direct correlation of esophageal motor abnormalities with spontaneously occurring chest pain episodes.[48,49] Further, ambulatory 24-hour esophageal manometry, which multiplies

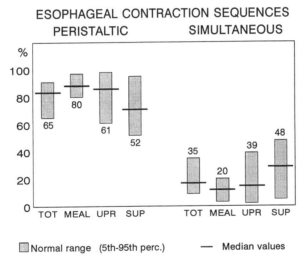

Fig. 2-17 Median values and normal range (5th to 95th percentiles) of percent of peristaltic and simultaneous esophageal contraction sequences recorded during 24-hour esophageal motility monitoring. Esophageal sequence (or wave) is defined as the presence of esophageal contractions in two adjacent recording sites, related to each other within 5 seconds. They are classified as a peristaltic progression if the peak-to-peak timing is ≥1 cm/sec between the two channels. In the normal subjects, 80% of esophageal waves are peristaltic during meals. The percentage of simultaneous waves normally decreases during meals and increases during sleep. Numbers represent the lower and upper limits of normal. TOT = total period of the test; UPR = daytime period excluding meals; SUP = sleep period. (From DeMeester TR, Costantini M. Esophageal function tests. In Pearson FG, ed. Esophageal Surgery. New York: Churchill Livingstone, 1995 [in press].)

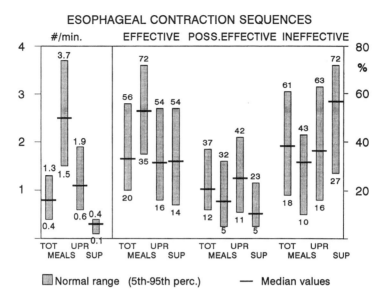

Fig. 2-18 Median values and normal range for the frequency of esophageal contraction sequences during different periods of the 24-hour esophageal motility monitoring, with the corresponding classification of the contraction sequences according to the percentage that are effective, possibly effective, and ineffective in the clearance of a liquid bolus. An effective sequence or wave is defined as the presence of peristaltic contractions in all three esophageal levels, with amplitude >20, 25, and 30 mm Hg, respectively, for 15, 10, and 5 cm above the LES. Possibly effective waves are those with peristaltic contractions in all three levels, with amplitude below the above values, but >15 mm Hg. Ineffective waves are defined as those with simultaneous, mixed, interrupted, or dropped contractions. Again, an increase in the frequency of esophageal waves is normally observed during meals, during which time they are also most effective. The maximum percentage of ineffective contractions is recorded during sleep, during a time when frequency is also decreased. Numbers represent the lower and upper limits of normal. TOT = total period of the test; UPR = daytime period excluding meals; SUP = sleep period. (From DeMeester TR, Costantini M. Esophageal function tests. In Pearson FG, ed. Esophageal Surgery. New York: Churchill Livingstone, 1995 [in press].)

the number of esophageal contractions available for analysis and provides an opportunity to assess esophageal motor function in a variety of physiologic situations such as sleep, awake, and meal periods, has been applied to the study of esophageal motor disorders to increase the accuracy and dependability of the measurement and classification.[50] However, ambulatory 24-hour manometry has been particularly useful in the evaluation of esophageal motility in patients with GERD.[51,52] In fact, primary esophageal motor activity is the most important factor in the clearance of refluxed gastric contents. Simultaneous manometry and video fluoroscopy showed that in the distal esophagus peristaltic contractions with a minimum amplitude of 30 mm Hg are required to completely occlude the esophageal lumen and propel a bolus.[5] This is confirmed by studies using combined esophageal pH and motility monitoring, which showed that the duration of a spontaneously occurring reflux episode is directly related to the frequency of peristaltic esophageal contractions

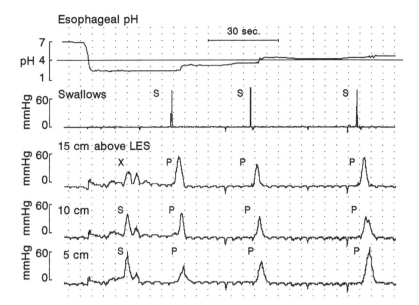

Fig. 2-19 Record of 24-hour ambulatory esophageal motility and pH monitoring in a normal subject. A gastroesophageal reflux episode (top tracing) was rapidly cleared by two swallows (*S*, second tracing) that initiated effective contractions (*P*) in the esophageal body (primary peristalsis). Note that the first contraction sequence (*S*) after the occurrence of the reflux was not initiated by a swallow and represents a secondary contraction that appeared to be simultaneous. The combined esophageal motility and pH monitoring with swallowing detection revealed that secondary contractions actually play little role in esophageal clearance. X = low-amplitude contraction. (From DeMeester TR, Costantini M. Esophageal function tests. In Pearson FG, ed. Esophageal Surgery. New York: Churchill Livingstone, 1995 [in press].)

with sufficient amplitude after the onset of the reflux episode.[53] Further, it has recently been shown that clearance of reflux episodes is mainly related to primary peristalsis following a pharyngeal swallowing[54] (Fig. 2-19). This suggests that ambulatory esophageal motility monitoring allows evaluation of esophageal clearance function by assessing the prevalence of efficient esophageal contractions, that is, the peristaltic contractions with an amplitude above 30 mm Hg, over an entire circadian cycle.

Application of ambulatory 24-hour esophageal motility monitoring in a series of patients with increased esophageal acid exposure and various degrees of esophageal mucosal injury showed that esophageal contractility deteriorates with increasing severity of esophageal mucosal injury.[51] This appears to occur secondary to persistent reflux across a mechanically defective LES and results in a marked increase in the frequency of inefficient esophageal contractions during the supine, upright, and meal periods, particularly in patients with stricture or Barrett's esophagus. The compromised clearance activity in this situation prolongs esophageal exposure to refluxed gastric juice (Fig. 2-20), indicated by the increased frequency of reflux episodes lasting longer than 5 minutes in these patients. Thus a vicious cycle

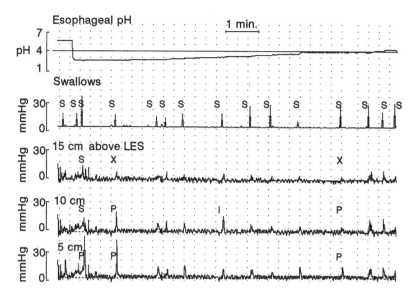

Fig. 2-20   Record of 24-hour ambulatory esophageal motility and pH monitoring in a patient with erosive esophagitis showing a gastroesophageal reflux episode (top tracing shows drop in pH from 6 to 2), with prolonged clearing time because of ineffective body motility. Repetitive swallows *(S)* elicited esophageal contractions of very low amplitude that on only a few occasions reached the threshold amplitude of 15 mm Hg to be recognized by the computer. P = peristaltic contractions; S = simultaneous contractions; X = low-amplitude contraction; I = isolated contraction. (From De-Meester TR, Costantini M. Esophageal function tests. In Pearson FG, ed. Esophageal Surgery. New York: Churchill Livingstone, 1995 [in press].)

is established. Deteriorated contractility also affects propulsion of swallowed food and, once lost, may not recover with treatment, even after a successful antireflux operation. A surgical correction of the underlying defect (i.e., the mechanically defective LES) early in the course of the disease is implicated. Once effective contractility has been lost, the surgical approach may have to be altered by using a repair with minimal outflow obstruction, that is, a partial fundoplication. Assessment of esophageal clearance function by ambulatory motility monitoring in patients with GERD helps to identify these patients with a greater degree of certainty than stationary motility.

AMBULATORY 24-HOUR pH MONITORING OF THE DISTAL ESOPHAGUS

Prior to the introduction of esophageal pH monitoring, an objective definition of GERD was difficult because the patient's history is not sufficiently accurate to precisely diagnose pathologic gastroesophageal reflux.[1] In addition, endoscopic or histologic evidence of esophagitis identifies only a complication of increased esophageal exposure to gastric juice and cannot be used to define the presence of disease because approximately 40% of patients have abnormally high exposure of the esophagus to gastric juice without complications.[15] To define a disease by the presence of its complications makes no sense. Defining GERD as an increased exposure of the esophageal lumen to gastric juice provides a means to objectively diagnose the presence of disease. This is possible with the use of ambulatory esophageal pH monitoring, first described by Miller[55] in 1964. Ten years later, it was used to quantitate the actual time the esophageal mucosa was exposed to gastric juice.[56] Subsequently, it has been shown that the test also assesses the ability of the esophagus to clear the refluxed acid juice and documents the relationship between esophageal exposure to gastric juice and the symptoms experienced by the patient.[14]

The test is performed using a small pH electrode passed transnasally and placed 5 cm above the upper border of the LES as measured by manometry. Different probes are available, but bipolar glass electrodes are preferred because of their greater reliability[57] and the elimination of an external reference electrode. The electrode is connected to an external portable solid-state data logger and pH values of the distal esophagus are continuously recorded, at 4-second intervals, for 24 hours, a complete circadian cycle. Pre- and postcalibration of the system at pH 1.0 and 7.0 is important to exclude electrode drift over the period of the study. All medications interfering with the gastrointestinal activity (especially H_2 blockers) must be discontinued at least 48 hours before beginning the test. A washout period of at least 1 week, and in some situations up to 4 weeks, is necessary in patients treated with omeprazole because of its long-lasting action.[58]

The test is performed on an outpatient basis, preferably while the subject is attending to normal activities. The patient is requested to remain in the upright position (or sitting) during the day, to lie down only at night while sleeping, and to ingest two meals at the usual times. The diet is standardized to exclude food and beverages with a pH value of less than 5.0 and greater than 6.0. Only water is allowed between meals. Patients are also instructed to keep a detailed diary of their symptoms during the study to correlate them with episodes of gastroesophageal reflux. They are asked to record the time when retiring for the night and when rising in the morning. Fig. 2-21 shows a typical esophageal pH monitoring trace in a healthy subject and in a patient with GERD.

It is important to emphasize that 24-hour pH esophageal monitoring should *not* be considered a test for reflux but rather a measurement of the esophageal exposure to gastric juice, that is, the amount of time the esophagus pH is below a given threshold during the 24-hour period. This expression, however, does not reflect how the exposure has occurred. For example, it could have occurred in a few long or several short reflux episodes. Consequently, two other measurements are necessary: the frequency of the reflux episodes and their duration. Esophageal exposure to gastric juice is best assessed by the following measurements: (1) cumulative time that the esophageal pH is below a chosen threshold, expressed as the percent of the total, upright, and supine position monitored time; (2) frequency of reflux episodes below a given threshold, expressed as number of reflux episodes per 24 hours; (3) duration of the episodes, expressed as the number of episodes lasting longer than 5 minutes per 24 hours; and (4) the time in minutes of the longest episode recorded.[56] Normal values for these components of the 24-hour record at each whole number

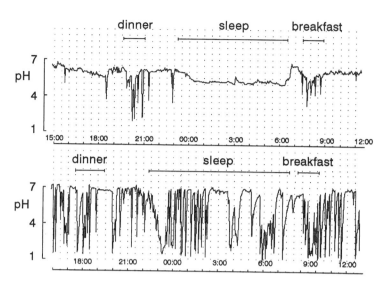

Fig. 2-21   Record of 24-hour pH monitoring of the distal esophagus in a healthy subject *(top)* and in a patient with esophagitis *(bottom)*. Physiologic gastroesophageal reflux episodes occur in a normal subject mainly in the upright position and after meals. The patient's record shows the presence of an increased number of reflux episodes, both in the upright and supine position, some of them with prolonged clearing time. (From DeMeester TR, Costantini M. Esophageal function tests. In Pearson FG, ed. Esophageal Surgery. New York: Churchill Livingstone, 1995 [in press].)

pH threshold were derived from 50 asymptomatic control subjects. The upper limits of normal were established at the 95th percentile.[59] If a symptomatic patient's values are outside the 95th percentile of normal subjects, he or she is considered abnormal for the component being measured. Most centers use pH 4 as the threshold. Using this threshold, there is a uniformity of normal values for these components from centers throughout the world.[60,61] This indicates that esophageal acid exposure can be quantitated and that normal individuals have similar values despite nationality or dietary habits. The normal values for these components obtained in 50 healthy volunteers are shown in Table 2-7. The upper limits of normality in other series are also shown for comparison.

To combine the results of the components into one expression of the overall esophageal acid exposure below a pH threshold, a pH score can be calculated using the standard deviation of the mean of each of the components measured in the 50 normal subjects as a weighing factor.[59] The calculated score for each component is added to obtain a composite score for each of the 50 normal subjects and the upper level of a normal score is established at the 95th percentile. The upper limits of normal for the composite score for each whole number pH threshold are shown in Table 2-8. The median and 95th percentile for the composite score for each whole number pH threshold can also be expressed graphically (Fig. 2-22). Personal computer–compatible software to perform this function is available (Gastrosoft, Inc., Irving, Tex.).

Table 2-7   Normal values for ambulatory pH monitoring in 50 healthy volunteers

	Mean	Standard Deviation	Median	Minimum	Maximum	95% Percentile
Total time pH <4 (%)	1.51	1.4	1.2	0	6.0	4.45
Upright time pH <4 (%)	2.2	2.3	1.6	0	9.3	8.4
Supine time pH <4 (%)	0.6	1.0	0.1	0	4.0	3.5
No. of episodes	19.0	12.8	16.0	2.0	56.0	46.9
No. of episodes >5 min	0.8	1.2	0	0	5.0	3.5
Longest episode (min)	6.7	7.9	4.0	0	46.0	19.8
Composite score	6.0	4.4	5.0	0.4	18.0	14.7

Table 2-8   95th percentile of the composite score for various pH thresholds

pH Threshold	95th Percentile
pH <1	14.2
pH <2	17.4
pH <3	14.1
pH <4	14.7
pH <5	15.8
pH >7	14.9
pH >8	8.5

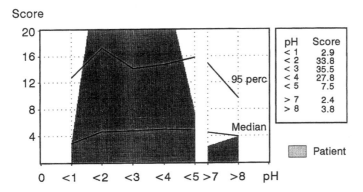

Fig. 2-22   The composite pH score is used to express the overall results for esophageal pH monitoring for the pH thresholds shown. The lower black line represents the median score and the upper black line represents the 95th percentile of 50 normal subjects. The gray area represents the score of a patient with increased esophageal acid exposure using the various pH thresholds as an indicator of reflux. The scores for esophageal acid exposure <4, <3, and <2 are abnormal.

Receiver-operator characteristic (ROC) analysis, in which sensitivity is plotted against specificity for a given test, was applied to each of the parameters and to the composite score using pH 4 as the threshold. Both total percent time below pH 4 and the composite score were found to have optimal specificity and sensitivity.[62] The normal pH data from three major centers in the United States have recently been combined to allow evaluation of the effects of age and gender on esophageal acid exposure. Men were found to have more physiologic reflux than women.[61] Consequently, when using the percent time below pH 4 as the criterion for identifying abnormal acid exposure, gender must be considered, particularly in those patients with borderline test results. The composite scoring system was found to be unaffected by gender.

The detection of increased esophageal exposure to acid gastric juice is more dependable than that of alkaline gastric juice. The latter is suggested by an alkaline exposure above pH 7 or 8. Increased exposure in this pH range can be caused by abnormal calibration of the pH recorder, the presence of dental infection that increases salivary pH, the presence of esophageal obstruction that results in static pools of saliva with an increase in pH secondary to bacterial overgrowth, or the presence of regurgitation of alkaline gastric juice into the esophagus.[63] Combined

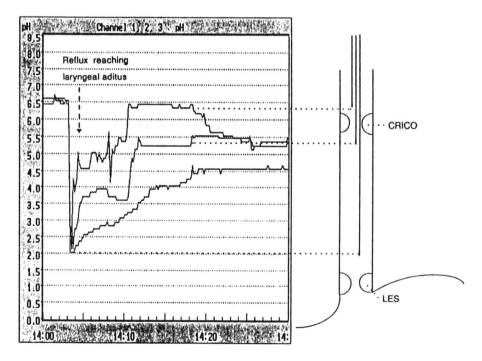

Fig. 2-23   Triple esophageal pH monitoring. Acid gastroesophageal reflux reaching the level of the laryngeal aditus provides good evidence of the association of GERD and respiratory symptoms. (From Bremner RM, DeMeester TR. Pre- and postoperative assessments in gastroesophageal reflux disease. In Scarpignato C, Galmiche JP, eds. Frontiers in Gastrointestinal Research, vol. 22. Functional Evaluation of Esophageal Disease. Basel: Karger, 1994, pp 260-287.)

gastric and esophageal pH monitoring in this situation increases the reliability of the test in detecting alkaline reflux.[64] Further, the new technology of 24-hour monitoring of bilirubin concentration seems to overcome these limitations and allows reliable detection of reflux of duodenal contents into the esophagus.[65]

An analysis of the pH data of patients with GERD using the time of exposure to different pH intervals (pH 0 to 1, 1 to 2, 2 to 3, etc.) has shown that increased exposure to a pH of 0 to 2 and 7 to 8 was associated with mucosal injury (esophagitis, stricture, or Barrett's esophagus) in 89% of patients.[66] In a different group of patients,[67] the amount of acid exposure to a pH of 1.5 to 2.5 in the supine position was able to predict the severity of the mucosal damage in 75% of patients. Therefore, 24-hour esophageal pH monitoring is not only useful in diagnosing the presence of GERD, but is also a useful test in predicting the presence of complications of the disease.

In patients with symptoms of chronic cough, hoarseness, or aspiration, placement of an additional pH electrode in the proximal part of the esophagus or pharynx can be helpful.[68,69] If reflux episodes reach to the proximal esophagus or pharynx, and a temporary relationship between these reflux episodes and the onset of the symptom can be documented, gastroesophageal reflux can be assumed to be the cause of the patient's complaint[70] (Fig. 2-23).

24-HOUR MONITORING OF ESOPHAGEAL EXPOSURE TO DUODENAL JUICE

The relevance of reflux of duodenal contents into the esophagus in determining the most severe grade of esophagitis has been outlined in the past.[71,72] Early clinical studies used the percentage of time the pH was above 7 on ambulatory esophageal pH monitoring as an indirect method of identifying esophageal exposure to duodenal contents. However, only the most severe episodes of duodenogastric and gastroesophageal reflux were detectable.

An ambulatory monitoring system has recently been developed that allows spectrophotometric measurements of luminal bilirubin concentration.[73] Using bilirubin as a natural marker, the time of esophageal exposure to duodenal contents can be measured. In the absence of carotene and serum lipids, the bilirubin concentration in a solution can be directly measured by spectrophotometry based on specific absorption at a wavelength of 453 nm. According to Beer's law, absorbance *(A)* is the logarithm of the ratio between the intensity of light transmitted *(I°)* through a solution containing an absorbing substance and the intensity of light transmitted *(I)* in the absence of the absorbing substance:

$$A = \log (I°/I)$$

The apparatus used to measure the presence of bilirubin consists of a portable opticoelectronic data logger, weighing 1200 gm, which can be strapped to the patient's side, and a fiberoptic probe, which can be passed transnasally and positioned anywhere in the lumen of the foregut (Bilitec 2000; Prodotec Srl, Florence, Italy; and Synectics Medical, Dallas, Tex.). The spectrophotometric probes are 3 mm in

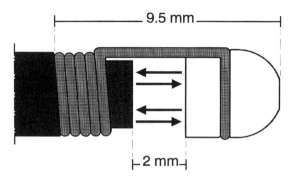

Fig. 2-24   The tip of the fiberoptic probe for the assessment of bilirubin concentration, with a 2 mm space for sampling. Fluid can easily move into and out of the space and the presence of bilirubin can be detected by its absorbance. (From Kauer WKH, Burdiles P, Ireland AP, Clark GWB, Peters JH, Bremner CG, DeMeester TR. Does duodenal juice reflux into the esophagus of patients with complication GERD? Evaluation of a fiberoptic sensor for bilirubin. Am J Surg 169:98-104, 1995.)

diameter and 140 cm in length and contain 30 plastic optical fibers, each 250 nm in diameter, bonded together and covered with biocompatible polyurethane. Two plugs connect 50% of the optic fibers to the light-emitting diodes and 50% to the receiving photo diode. The tip of the probe contains a 2 mm space for sampling (Fig. 2-24). Fluid and blenderized solids can easily flow through the space and their bilirubin concentration can be measured. The probes are flexible, durable, easy to sterilize, and reusable. The optoelectronic unit acts simultaneously as a light signal generator, a data processor, and a data storage device. Further, the unit has two channels allowing dual measurement with two probes if desired. The light source for each channel is provided by two light-emitting diodes that emit a 470 nm signal light (blue spectrum) and a 565 nm reference light (green spectrum). Reference and signal light-emitting diodes are stimulated alternately for a duration of 0.5 second. To avoid fluctuations in the source, the final 20 milliseconds of each pulse are used for signal processing. Optical signals reflected back from the probe are converted to electrical impulses by a photo diode. This electrical signal is then amplified and processed within the data logger. Absorbance readings are averaged every two cycles. The system is capable of recording 225 individual absorbance values per hour and allows up to 30 hours of continuous monitoring.

Recent in vitro and in vivo validation studies[65,73] showed that spectrophotometry based on absorption at a wavelength of 453 nm is specific for bilirubin and that the absorbance spectrum is sufficient to detect bilirubin throughout human physiologic ranges. Further, the measurements are highly reproducible despite pH changes caused by environment or food intake. In addition, in a clinical study an absorbance threshold of 0.14 was found to be a reliable threshold to differentiate healthy subjects from reflux patients. Patients with Barrett's esophagus showed the highest individual values and a significantly higher exposure than controls when the esophageal pH was <4 or between 4 and 7, which are ranges in which pH monitoring cannot detect alkaline reflux (pH >7).[65]

Therefore, this test is a very useful and reliable complementary tool to esophageal pH monitoring in the investigation of patients with foregut symptoms. The combination of pH and bilirubin esophageal monitoring will further our understanding and improve our care of patients with GERD.

AMBULATORY 24-HOUR GASTRIC pH MONITORING

Functional disorders of the esophagus are not often confined to the esophagus alone, but are associated with functional disorders of the rest of the foregut (i.e., stomach and duodenum). Abnormalities of gastric emptying,[74,75] gastric dilation, increased intragastric pressure,[76] and increased gastric acid secretion,[77] can be responsible for increased esophageal exposure to gastric juice. Reflux of alkaline duodenal juice, including bile salts and pancreatic enzymes, is involved in the pathogenesis of esophagitis and the complication of stricture and Barrett's esophagus.[71,72] Gastric causes should therefore be considered in patients with increased esophageal exposure to gastric juice on ambulatory pH monitoring and a normal LES on manometry. Gastric analysis may be required to exclude hypersecretion and gastric emptying studies should be performed if delayed emptying is suspected. Further, an *o*-diisopropyl iminodiacetic acid (DISIDA) scan with cholecystokinin (CCK) stimulation may be required to investigate a suspected duodenogastric reflux. All these situations can be investigated by ambulatory 24-hour gastric pH monitoring.

Ambulatory 24-hour gastric pH monitoring is performed in a way similar to esophageal pH monitoring and often the two tests are performed together, with combined bipolar glass electrodes positioned 5 cm below the lower border of the LES. The interpretation of gastric pH recordings is, however, more difficult than that of esophageal recordings because the gastric pH environment is determined by a complex interplay of acid and mucous secretion, ingested food, swallowed saliva, regurgitated duodenal, pancreatic, and biliary secretions, and the effectiveness of the mixing and evacuation of the chyme. In this connection, a set of parameters describing the circadian gastric pH pattern has been developed, which allows the quantitation of duodenogastric reflux and gastric acid secretion based on the circadian pH record and which may be helpful in the assessment of gastric emptying disorders.

To quantitate alkaline duodenogastric reflux,[78] the gastric pH record is divided into the upright period, the supine period, the prandial pH plateau period, and the postprandial pH decline period. For each of these periods the following parameters are calculated:
1. The pH frequency distribution, that is, the percentage time the gastric pH was at the pH interval 0 to 1, 1 to 2, 2 to 3, 3 to 4, 4 to 5, 5 to 6, 6 to 7, and above 7.
2. The frequency of pH changes, that is, the incidence of pH movements from a lower into a higher pH interval.
3. The duration of pH exposure expressed as the longest time the pH remained at a pH interval during the monitoring period.

4. Duration-frequency of pH exposure expressed as the number of times the pH remained at a pH interval for longer than 5 minutes.

Using discriminant analysis, a scoring system based on 16 of these parameters can completely differentiate the gastric pH profile of normal volunteers from patients with classic duodenogastric reflux disease. When applied prospectively, this scoring system was superior to DISIDA scanning with CCK stimulation in the diagnosis of excessive duodenogastric reflux and detected the disease with a sensitivity of 90% and a specificity of 100%.[78]

Ambulatory 24-hour gastric monitoring can also be used to evaluate the gastric secretory state of the patient. This is of particular value since the role of gastric acid secretion in the pathogenesis of GERD is well documented and it has recently been shown that 28% of patients with objectively proved GERD had gastric hypersecretion.[77] To do so, the frequency distribution and the cumulative frequency distribution graphs of the pH data of the patient are plotted against the range (5th to 95th percentiles) of the same graphs obtained in 50 healthy volunteers (Fig. 2-25). In our experience, this approach correlates well with the data obtained by traditional gastric secretion studies.[79]

Evaluation of gastric emptying on the basis of the postprandial alkalinization of the gastric pH record is a new concept that evolved from multiple-probe gastric pH monitoring during gastric emptying studies with radiolabeled meals. These studies demonstrated a good correlation between the emptying of oatmeal and the duration of the postprandial plateau and decline phases of the gastric pH record.[79] A prolonged postprandial alkalinization of the pH in the corpus may therefore indicate delayed gastric emptying of solids.

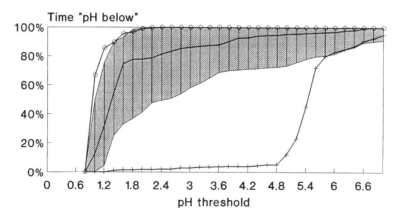

Fig. 2-25 Cumulative frequency distribution of recorded gastric pH values during the supine period. The shaded area represents the 5th and 95th percentiles of 50 healthy volunteers and the solid line shows the median. Patient M.G. (○) with a duodenal ulcer had a shift of the median values above the normal range, suggesting gastric acid hypersecretion. Patient B.C. (+) had a shift of the median values below the normal range, indicating hypochlorhydria. (From Stein HJ, DeMeester TR, Hinder RA. Outpatient physiologic testing and surgical management of foregut motility disorders. Curr Probl Surg 24:418-555, 1992.)

COMPLETE FOREGUT OUTPATIENT PHYSIOLOGIC MONITORING

The development of miniaturized pH electrodes, electronic pressure transducers, and fiberoptic probes and the introduction of portable digital data recorders with large storage capacities have recently made possible prolonged monitoring of luminal pH, bilirubin concentration, and motor activity of the foregut in an outpatient environment (see Fig. 2-15). Ambulatory 24-hour monitoring of foregut pH, motility, and bilirubin concentration overcomes the limitations of the standard tests classically used to assess foregut function. It allows the recording of foregut function under physiologic conditions over a complete circadian cycle. This increases the probability of recording disordered motility and episodes of spontaneous gastroesophageal or duodenogastric reflux. It allows quantitation of the observed abnormalities and their direct correlation with spontaneously occurring symptoms. With the use of modern solid-state recording technology and computerized reading, prolonged foregut monitoring over periods of 24 hours has become safe to perform and easy to analyze. Broad clinical application of this new technology will replace the series of laboratory tests classically required to thoroughly evaluate foregut function. This new technology puts tools into the surgeon's hand to evaluate complex foregut problems within the office and places surgical therapy of functional abnormalities of the foregut on a more scientific basis.

REFERENCES

1. Costantini M, Crookes PF, Bremner RM, Hoeft SF, Ehsan A, Peters JH, Bremner CG, De-Meester TR. Value of physiologic assessment of foregut symptoms in a surgical practice. Surgery 114:780-787, 1993.
2. DeMeester TR, Bonavina L, Iascone C, Courtney JV, Skinner DB. Chronic respiratory symptoms and occult gastroesophageal reflux. Ann Surg 211:337-345, 1990.
3. DeMeester TR, Costantini M. Esophageal function tests. In Pearson FG, ed. Esophageal Surgery. New York: Churchill Livingstone, 1995 (in press).
4. Hewson EG, Ott DJ, Dalton CB, Chen YM, Wu WC, Richter JE. Manometry and radiology: Complementary studies in the assessment of esophageal motility disorders. Gastroenterology 98:626-632, 1990.
5. Kahrilas PJ, Dodds WJ, Hogan WJ. Effect of peristaltic dysfunction on esophageal volume clearance. Gastroenterology 94:73-80, 1988.
6. Ott DJ. Radiology of the oropharynx and esophagus. In Castell DO, ed. The Esophagus. Boston: Little Brown, 1994, pp 41-88.
7. Ott DJ, Kelley TF, Chen MYM, Gelfand DW. Evaluation of the esophagus with a marshmallow bolus: Clarifying the cause of dysphagia. Gastrointest Radiol 16:1-4, 1991.
8. Dantas RO, Cook IJ, Dodds WJ, Kern MH, Lang IM, Brasseur JG. Biomechanics of cricopharyngeal bars. Gastroenterology 99:1269-1274, 1990.
9. Gelfand DW. Radiologic evaluation of the esophagus. In Orringer MB, ed. Shackelford's Surgery of the Alimentary Tract. Philadelphia: WB Saunders, 1991.
10. Orlando RC, Call DL, Bream CA. Achalasia and absent gastric air bubble. Ann Intern Med 88:60-61, 1978.
11. Kahrilas PJ, Dodds WJ, Hogan WJ, Kern M, Arndorfer RC, Reece A. Esophageal peristaltic dysfunction in peptic esophagitis. Gastroenterology 91:897-904, 1986.
12. Ott DJ. Radiology of esophageal function and gastroesophageal reflux disease. In Scarpignato C, Galmiche JP, eds. Frontiers in Gastrointestinal Research, vol. 22. Functional Evaluation in Esophageal Disease. Basel: Karger, 1994, pp 27-70.

13. Kahn KL, Kosecoff J, Chassin MR, Solomon DH, Brook RH. The use and misuse of upper gastrointestinal endoscopy. Ann Intern Med 109:664-670, 1988.
14. DeMeester TR, Wang CI, Wernly JA, Pellegrini CA, Little AG, Klementschitsch P, Bermudez G, Johnson LF, Skinner DB. Technique, indications and clinical use of 24-hour esophageal pH monitoring. J Thorac Cardiovasc Surg 79:656-670, 1980.
15. Fuchs KH, DeMeester TR, Albertucci M. Specificity and sensitivity of objective diagnosis of gastroesophageal reflux disease. Surgery 102:575-580, 1987.
16. Richter JE, Castell DO. Gastroesophageal reflux. Pathogenesis, diagnosis and treatment. Ann Intern Med 97:93-103, 1982.
17. Savary M, Miller G. The esophagus. In Handbook and Atlas of Endoscopy. Solothurn, Switzerland: Gassmann, 1978, p 135.
18. Tytgat GNJ, Tytgat SHAJ. Esophageal biopsy. In Scarpignato C, Galmiche JP, eds. Frontiers in Gastrointestinal Research, vol. 22. Functional Evaluation in Esophageal Disease. Basel: Karger, 1994, pp 13-26.
19. Streitz JM Jr, Williamson WA, Ellis FH Jr. Current concepts concerning the nature and treatment of Barrett's esophagus and its complications. Ann Thorac Surg 54:586-591, 1992.
20. Tytgat GNJ, Hameeteman W. The neoplastic potential of columnar-lined (Barrett's) esophagus. World J Surg 16:308-312, 1992.
21. Arndorfer RC, Stef JJ, Dodds WJ, Linehan JH, Hogan WJ. Improved infusion system for intraluminal esophageal manometry. Gastroenterology 73:23-27, 1977.
22. Dodds WJ, Hogan WJ, Stef JJ, Miller WN, Lydon SB, Arndorfer RC. A rapid pull-through technique for measuring lower esophageal sphincter pressure. Gastroenterology 68:437-443, 1975.
23. Winans CS, Harris LD. Quantitation of lower esophageal sphincter competence. Gastroenterology 52:773-778, 1967.
24. Welch RW, Drake ST. Normal lower esophageal sphincter pressure: A comparison of rapid vs. slow pull-through techniques. Gastroenterology 78:1446-1451, 1980.
25. Winans CS. Manometric asymmetry of the lower esophageal high-pressure zone. Am J Dig Dis 22:348-354, 1977.
26. Costantini M, Bremner RM, Hoeft SF, Crookes PF, DeMeester TR. The slow motorized pull-through: An improved technique to evaluate the lower esophageal sphincter. Gastroenterology 103:1407, 1992.
27. Stein HJ, DeMeester TR, Naspetti R, Jamieson J, Perry RE. Three-dimensional imaging of the lower esophageal sphincter in gastroesophageal reflux disease. Ann Surg 214:374-384, 1991.
28. Bombeck CT, Vas O, DeSalvo J, Donahue PE, Nyhus LM. Computerized axial manometry of the esophagus: A new method for the assessment of antireflux operation. Ann Surg 206:465-472, 1987.
29. Richter JE, Wu WC, Johns DM, Blackwell JN, Nelson JL III, Castell JA, Castell DO. Esophageal manometry in 95 healthy adult volunteers: Variability of pressure with age and frequency of "abnormal" contractions. Dig Dis Sci 32:583-592, 1987.
30. Costantini M, Bremner RM, Hoeft SF, Crookes PF, DeMeester TR. Normal esophageal motor function: A manometric study of 136 healthy subjects. Gastroenterology 103:1407, 1993.
31. Welch RW, Luckmann K, Ricks PM, Drake ST, Gates GA. Manometry of the normal upper esophageal sphincter and its alterations in laryngectomy. J Clin Invest 63:1036-1041, 1979.
32. Kahrilas PJ, Dodds WJ, Dent J, Logemann JA, Shaker R. Upper esophageal sphincter function during deglutition. Gastroenterology 95:52-62, 1988.
33. Crookes PF, Stein HJ, DeMeester TR. Stationary manometry of the esophageal body and upper esophageal sphincter. In Hinder RA, ed. Problems in General Surgery, vol. 9. Tests of Foregut Function, 1992, pp 39-61.
34. Kahrilas PJ, Dent J, Dodds WJ, Hogan WJ, Arndorfer RC. A method for continuous monitoring of the upper esophageal sphincter pressure. Dig Dis Sci 32:121-128, 1987.
35. Castell JA, Dalton CB, Castell DO. Pharyngeal and upper esophageal sphincter manometry in humans. Am J Physiol 258:G173-G178, 1990.
36. Hocking MP, Ryckman FC, Woodward ER. Achalasia mimicking peptic esophageal stricture. Am Surg 51:563-566, 1985.

37. Zaninotto G, Peserico A, Costantini M, Salvador L, Rondinone R, Roveran A, Piasentin G, Ancona E, Glorioso S, Merigliano S. Oesophageal motility and lower oesophageal sphincter competence in progressive systemic sclerosis and localized scleroderma. Scand J Gastroenterol 24:95-102, 1989.

38. Zaninotto G, DeMeester TR, Schwitzer W, Johansson K-E, Cheng SC. The lower esophageal sphincter in health and disease. Am J Surg 155:104-111, 1988.

39. Lieberman DA. Medical therapy for chronic reflux esophagitis: Long-term follow-up. Arch Intern Med 147:1717-1720, 1987.

40. Costantini M, Zaninotto G, Boccu' C, Anselmino M, Bagolin F, Nicoletti L, Merigliano S, Ancona E. Is the manometric finding of a defective lower esophageal sphincter clinically useful? Gut 35(S4):A182, 1994.

41. Costantini M, Zaninotto G, Anselmino M, Boccu' C, Nicoletti L, Bagolin F, Ancona E. Manometric evaluation of the lower esophageal sphincter in gastroesophageal reflux disease: A modern approach. Br J Surg 80:S62, 1993.

42. Joelsson BE, DeMeester TR, Skinner DB, Lafontaine E, Waters PF, O'Sullivan GC. The role of the esophageal body in the antireflux mechanism. Surgery 92:417-424, 1982.

43. Duranceau A, Lafontaine E, Taillfer R. Oropharyngeal dysphagia. In Jamieson GG, ed. Surgery of the Oesophagus. London: Churchill Livingstone, 1988.

44. Bonavina L, Khan NA, DeMeester TR. Pharyngoesophageal dysfunction. The role of cricopharyngeal myotomy. Arch Surg 120:541-549, 1985.

45. Cook IJ, Gabb M, Panagopoulos V, Jamieson GG, Dodds WJ, Dent J, Shearman DJ. Pharyngeal (Zenker's) diverticulum is a disorder of upper esophageal sphincter opening. Gastroenterology 103:1229-1235, 1992.

46. Dantas RO, Kern MK, Massey BT, Dodds WJ, Kahrilas PJ, Brasseur JG, Cook IJ, Lang IM. Effect of swallowed bolus variables on oral and pharyngeal phases of swallowing. Am J Physiol 258:G675-G681, 1990.

47. Bremner RM, Costantini M, Hoeft SF, Yasui A, Crookes PF, Shibberu H, Peters JH, Nicholas K, DeMeester TR. Manual verification of computer analysis of 24-hour esophageal motility. Biomed Instrum Technol 27:49-55, 1993.

48. Maas LC, Gordon RK, Penner D, Barkel D, Gordon S, Linert D, Petty D. 24-hour ambulatory manometry in diagnosis of esophageal motor disorders causing chest pain. South Med J 78:810-813, 1985.

49. Janssens J, Vantrappen G, Ghillebert G. 24-hour recording of esophageal pressure and pH in patients with noncardiac chest pain. Gastroenterology 90:1978-1984, 1986.

50. Eypasch EP, Stein HJ, DeMeester TR, Johansson K-E, Barlow AP, Schneider GT. A new technique to define and clarify esophageal motor disorders. Am J Surg 159:144-152, 1990.

51. Stein HJ, Eypasch EP, DeMeester TR, Smyrk TC, Attwood SEA. Circadian esophageal motor function in patients with gastroesophageal reflux disease. Surgery 108:769-778, 1990.

52. Stein HJ, DeMeester TR. Indications, technique and clinical use of ambulatory 24-hour esophageal motility monitoring in a surgical practice. Ann Surg 217:128-137, 1993.

53. Bumm R, Feussner H, Emde C. Interaction of gastroesophageal reflux and esophageal motility in healthy men undergoing combined 24-hour mano/pH-metry. In Little AG, Ferguson MK, Skinner DB, eds. Diseases of the Esophagus. Mount Kisco, N.Y.: Futura Publishing Co., 1990, pp 101-113.

54. Bremner RM, Hoeft SF, Costantini M, Crookes PF, Bremner CG, DeMeester TR. Pharyngeal swallowing: The major factor in clearance of esophageal reflux episodes. Ann Surg 218:364-370, 1993.

55. Miller FA. Utilization of inlying pH-probe for evaluation of acid-peptic diathesis. Arch Surg 89:199-203, 1964.

56. Johnson LF, DeMeester TR. Twenty-four hour pH monitoring of the distal esophagus. A quantitative measure of gastroesophageal reflux. Am J Gastroenterol 62:325-332, 1974.

57. McLauchlan G, Rawlings JM, Lucas ML, McCloy RF, Crean GP, McColl KEL. Electrodes for 24 hour pH monitoring: A comparative study. Gut 28:935-939, 1987.

58. Marks IN, Young GO, Winter T, Zak J. Duration of acid inhibition after withdrawal of omeprazole treatment in D.U. patients in remission. S Afr Med J 82:42A, 1992.

59. DeMeester TR. Prolonged oesophageal pH monitoring. In Read NW, ed. Gastrointestinal Motility: Which Test? Petersfield, England: Wrightson Biomedical, 1989, pp 41-51.

60. Emde C, Garner A, Blum A. Technical aspects of intraluminal pH-metry in man: Current status and recommendations. Gut 23:1177-1188, 1987.

61. Richter JE, Bradley LA, DeMeester TR, Wu WC. Normal 24-hour pH values. Influence of study center, pH electrodes, age and gender. Dig Dis Sci 37:849-856, 1992.

62. Jamieson J, Stein HJ, DeMeester TR, Bonavina L, Schwizer W, Hinder RA, Albertucci M, Cheng S-C. Ambulatory 24-hour esophageal pH monitoring: Normal values, optimal thresholds, specificity, sensitivity and reproducibility. Am J Gastroenterol 87:1102-1111, 1992.

63. Stein HJ, DeMeester TR. Integrated ambulatory foregut monitoring in patients with functional foregut disorders. In Nyhus LM, ed. Surgery Annual. Part 1, vol. 24. Norwalk, Conn.: Appleton & Lange, 1992, pp 161-180.

64. Mattioli S, Pilotti V, Felice V, Lazzari A, Zanolli R, Bacchi LB, Loria P, Tripodi A, Gozzetti G. Ambulatory 24-hour pH monitoring of esophagus, fundus and antrum. A new technique for simultaneous study of gastroesophageal and duodenogastric reflux. Dig Dis Sci 35:929-938, 1990.

65. Kauer WKH, Burdiles P, Ireland AP, Clark GWB, Peters JH, Bremner CG, DeMeester TR. Does duodenal juice reflux into the esophagus of patients with complicated GERD? Evaluation of a fiberoptic sensor for bilirubin. Am J Surg 169:98-104, 1995.

66. Bremner RM, Crookes PF, DeMeester TR, Peters JH, Stein HJ. Concentration of refluxed acid and esophageal mucosal injury. Am J Surg 164:522-527, 1992.

67. Zaninotto G, Costantini M, DiMario F, Rugge M, Baffa R, Dal Santo PL, Germana' B, Naccarato R, Ancona E. Oesophagitis and pH of the refluxate: An experimental and clinical study. Br J Surg 79:161-164, 1992.

68. Jacob P, Kahrilas PJ, Herzon G. Proximal esophageal pH-metry in patients with "reflux laryngitis." Gastroenterology 100:305-310, 1991.

69. Patti MG, Debas HT, Pellegrini CA. Clinical and functional characterization of high gastroesophageal reflux. Am J Surg 165:163-168, 1993.

70. Bremner RM, DeMeester TR. Pre- and postoperative assessments in gastroesophageal reflux disease. In Scarpignato C, Galmiche JP, eds. Frontiers in Gastrointestinal Research, vol. 22. Functional Evaluation in Esophageal Disease. Basel: Karger, 1994, pp 260-287.

71. Stein HJ, Barlow AP, DeMeester TR, Hinder RA. Complications of gastroesophageal reflux disease: Role of the lower esophageal sphincter, esophageal acid and acid/alkaline exposure, and duodenogastric reflux. Ann Surg 216:35-43, 1992.

72. Attwood SEA, DeMeester TR, Bremner CG, Barlow AP, Hinder RA. Alkaline gastroesophageal reflux: Implications in the development of complications in Barrett's columnar-lined lower esophagus. Surgery 106:764-770, 1989.

73. Bechi P, Pucciani F, Baldini F, Cosi F, Falciai R, Mazzanti R, Castagnoli A, Passeri A, Boscherini S. Long-term ambulatory enterogastric reflux monitoring: Validation of a new fiberoptic technique. Dig Dis Sci 38:1297-1306, 1993.

74. McCallum RW, Berkowitz DM, Lerner E. Gastric emptying in patients with gastroesophageal acid reflux. Dig Dis Sci 26:993-998, 1981.

75. Schwizer W, Hinder RA, DeMeester TR. Does delayed gastric emptying contribute to gastroesophageal reflux disease? Am J Surg 157:74-81, 1989.

76. Bonavina L, Evander A, DeMeester TR, Walter B, Cheng SC, Palazzo L, Concannon JL. Length of the distal esophageal sphincter and competency of the cardia. Am J Surg 151:25-34, 1986.

77. Barlow AP, DeMeester TR, Ball CS, Eypasch EP. The significance of the gastric secretory state in gastroesophageal reflux disease. Arch Surg 124:937-940, 1989.

78. Fuchs KH, DeMeester TR, Hinder RA, Stein HJ, Barlow AP, Gupta NC. Computerized identification of pathologic duodenogastric reflux using 24-hour gastric pH monitoring. Ann Surg 213:13-20, 1991.

79. Stein HJ, DeMeester TR, Hinder RA. Outpatient physiologic testing and surgical management of foregut motility disorders. Curr Probl Surg 24:418-555, 1992.

3

Tailored Antireflux Surgery

Jeffrey H. Peters, M.D. • *Werner K.H. Kauer*, M.D.
Tom R. DeMeester, M.D.

Antireflux surgery is different from the surgery to extirpate a diseased organ whose function is of no concern since it will be destroyed with its removal. Rather, antireflux surgery is designed to improve the function of an organ that will remain in the patient, that is, to provide complete and permanent relief of all symptoms and complications of gastroesophageal reflux secondary to an incompetent cardia. Successful surgery for antireflux disease requires tailoring of the surgical approach to the underlying physiology. Options include open and laparoscopic Nissen fundoplication, transthoracic approaches, partial fundoplications, such as the Belsey Mark IV, and esophageal lengthening procedures. Poor results are frequently based on an inappropriate procedure performed without consideration of underlying physiologic and anatomic abnormalities.

Most patients with gastroesophageal reflux disease (GERD) are treated medically for years (Fig. 3-1) and, at the time the patient is referred for surgery, the dis-

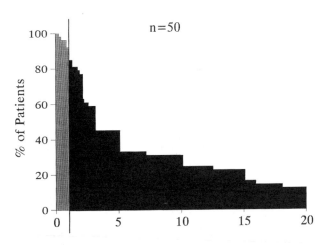

Fig. 3-1 Years of medical treatment in 50 patients referred for antireflux surgery. The mean time patients were treated medically prior to referral for surgical therapy was 4.5 years.

ease has often progressed to include functional and anatomic foregut alterations. Abnormalities of esophageal motility,[1] shortening of esophageal length, and the presence of a stricture or Barrett's metaplasia[2] are common. Antireflux surgery in this setting is particularly challenging, and when adjustments are not made for these abnormalities, the results can be less than satisfactory.

Antireflux surgery in patients with end-stage reflux disease often results in a high percentage of unsatisfactory results compared to patients with early disease.[3-6] Failure to use a tailored approach resulted in a long-term outcome of only 65% with good or excellent results. Salama and Lamont[4] reported that the clinical success of a Belsey fundoplication was 90% in patients with no esophagitis compared to 50% in patients with grade IV esophagitis or stricture. Similar results were pointed out by Skinner and Belsey[7] in their original description of the Belsey partial fundoplication in which a 40% recurrence rate was reported in patients who had esophageal stricture and shortening. Appropriate physiologic assessment prior to antireflux surgery becomes particularly important with the growing enthusiasm for minimally invasive techniques. Widespread application of laparoscopic Nissen fundoplication in all patients without objective assessment of deficits in esophageal length or function will likely lead to poor results in a significant number of patients with advanced disease.

PATIENT ASSESSMENT PRIOR TO THE OPERATION

Body habitus. Patients who are judged clinically to be obese are best approached through the chest to maximize surgical exposure.

Esophageal motility. Esophageal manometry should be performed in all patients prior to antireflux surgery.[8] Contraction amplitudes below the 5th percentile of normal at the same level of the esophagus are considered a failed contraction. Contraction velocities between two contraction peaks of 20 cm/sec or more are considered to be simultaneous rather than peristaltic. Using these definitions, failure of esophageal body function can be identified by the presence of a contraction amplitude below 20 mm Hg in one or more of the three lowest 5 cm esophageal segments or a prevalence of more than 20% simultaneous waves through these segments.

Endoscopy. Fiberoptic endoscopic examination is used to measure the position of the diaphragmatic crura, the location and distinctiveness of the squamocolumnar junction, and the presence of mucosal injury. Esophagitis is scored as grade I for an erythematous and friable mucosa, grade II for linear erosions, and grade III for deeper and wider linear erosions with islands of edematous mucosa between erosive furrows. Grade I esophagitis is considered subjective and should not be included as a complication for the purposes of procedure selection. An esophageal stricture is defined by the inability to pass a 36 F endoscope with ease. The diagnosis of Barrett's esophagus is made when histologic examination confirms specialized columnar-type epithelium above the anatomic gastroesophageal junction.

Esophageal length. Esophageal length can be assessed using video radiographic contrast studies and endoscopic findings. The esophageal length is considered too short for an abdominal approach if there is a hiatal hernia that fails to reduce in the upright position on the video barium esophagram, or if there is greater than 5 cm measured on endoscopy between the diaphragmatic crura, identified by having the patient sniff, and the gastroesophageal junction.

SELECTION OF PATIENTS FOR ANTIREFLUX SURGERY

Many internists and surgeons are reluctant to advise surgery in the absence of demonstrable esophagitis. However, antireflux surgery can be considered in a symptomatic patient provided the disease process has been objectively documented by 24-hour pH monitoring, particularly in patients who have become dependent on therapy with proton pump inhibitors.[9] Indeed, investigations of the natural history of GERD in the absence of esophagitis have demonstrated return of symptoms in the majority of patients following cessation of medical therapy.[10]

An incompetent lower esophageal sphincter (LES) is a significant factor predicting failure of medical therapy. Lieberman[11] compared symptomatic relapse in patients on long-term medical therapy. Patients with a mechanically incompetent LES (mean pressure, 4.9 mm Hg) did not respond well to medical therapy and usually developed recurrent symptoms within 1 to 2 years of the onset of therapy.[11] This study suggests that patients with deficient LES do not respond well to medical therapy, often relapse, and should be considered for an antireflux operation, regardless of the presence or absence of endoscopic esophagitis. If the LES is normal, evidence of gastric acid hypersecretion or delayed gastric emptying should be sought. We are cautious about performing fundoplication in patients with a normal LES. Such patients are often "upright" refluxers who are chronic air swallowers and do not do as well following antireflux surgery.

Young patients with documented reflux disease and a defective LES are also excellent candidates for antireflux surgery. They invariably require long-term medical therapy for control of their symptoms and many go on to develop complications of the disease. Furthermore, Coley et al.[12] have shown a cost advantage for surgery over medical therapy in patients younger than 49 years of age.

Endoscopic esophagitis in a symptomatic patient with a mechanically defective LES should raise the question of surgical therapy. These patients are prone to a relapse of their symptoms while receiving medical therapy.[13] Esophagitis is visualized endoscopically and usually classified by some modification of Savary and Miller's grading system.[14] In addition, the severity of the esophagitis is useful as a predictor for response to medical therapy.[15] Reports of the response rates of erosive esophagitis to medical treatment have been less than satisfactory. Hetzel et al.[15] reported a 97% healing rate of grades I and II esophagitis after 4 weeks of treatment with 40 mg omeprazole daily, but only 88% and 44% of grades III and IV, respectively, healed. If the patient responds symptomatically to medical therapy, but endoscopic esophagitis persists, surgery should be performed. Without surgery, these patients can progress to Barrett's esophagus and esophageal body function may deteriorate while on therapy.[16]

The development of a stricture in a patient with a mechanically defective sphincter represents a failure of medical therapy and is an indication for a surgical antireflux procedure. In addition, a stricture is usually associated with loss of esophageal contractility.[17] Prior to surgery, a malignant etiology of the stricture should be excluded and the stricture progressively dilated up to a 60 F bougie. When fully dilated, the relief of dysphagia is evaluated and esophageal manometry is performed to determine the adequacy of peristalsis in the distal esophagus. If dysphagia is relieved and the amplitude of esophageal contractions is adequate, an antireflux procedure should be performed. If the amplitude of esophageal contractions is poor, caution should be exercised in performing an antireflux procedure with a complete fundoplication and a partial fundoplication should be considered.

Barrett's columnar-lined esophagus is almost always associated with a severe mechanical defect of the LES and often poor contractility of the esophageal body.[18,19] Patients with Barrett's esophagus are at risk because of a progression of the mucosal abnormality in the esophagus, formation of a stricture, hemorrhage from a Barrett's ulcer, and the development of adenocarcinoma.[20] A surgical antireflux procedure may arrest the progression of the disease, heal ulceration, and resolve strictures.[21] If severe dysplasia or intramucosal carcinoma is found on mucosal biopsies, an esophageal resection should be done.[22]

FACTORS TO CONSIDER PRIOR TO ANTIREFLUX SURGERY

Prior to proceeding with an antireflux operation, several factors should be evaluated. First, the propulsive force of the body of the esophagus should be evaluated by esophageal manometry to determine if it has sufficient power to propel a bolus of food through a newly reconstructed valve[23] (Fig. 3-2). Esophageal body motor

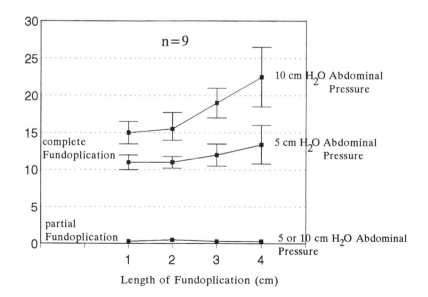

Fig. 3-2 Measurements of esophageal outflow resistance in adynamic cadaveric esophagogastric specimens. Outflow resistance varies depending on the degree and length of fundoplication (Belsey, Nissen).

function is commonly altered with advanced stages of GERD[1] (Fig. 3-3). Patients with normal peristaltic contractions have a good result after a 360-degree Nissen fundoplication. When peristalsis is absent, severely disordered, or the amplitude of the contraction is below 20 mm Hg, the Belsey two thirds partial fundoplication is the procedure of choice.[24]

Second, anatomic shortening of the esophagus can compromise the ability to do an adequate repair without tension and lead to an increased incidence of break-

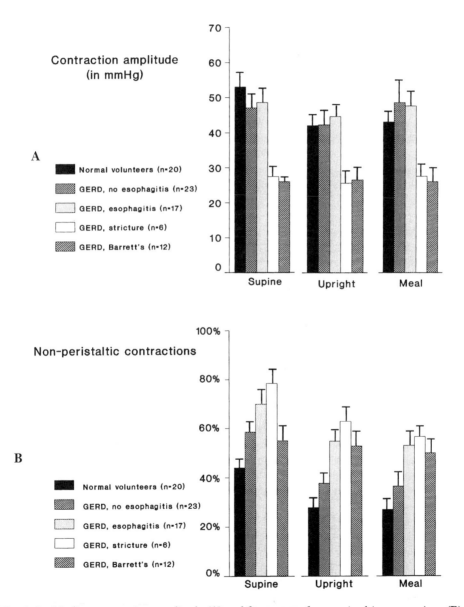

Fig. 3-3   Median contraction amplitude **(A)** and frequency of nonperistaltic contractions **(B)** on 24-hour ambulatory esophageal motility monitoring in patients with GERD and various degrees of mucosal injury. (From Stein HJ, Eypasch EP, DeMeester TR, et al. Circadian esophageal motor function in patients with gastroesophageal reflux disease. Surgery 108:773, 1990.)

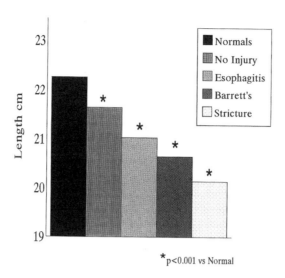

Fig. 3-4 Length of esophagus in patients with GERD compared to normal subjects. Esophageal length progressively shortens as complications of the disease become more severe.

down or thoracic displacement of the repair (Fig. 3-4). Esophageal shortening is identified radiographically by a sliding hiatal hernia that will not reduce in the upright position, or is more than 5 cm long when measured between the diaphragmatic crura and gastroesophageal junction on endoscopy. In the presence of a short esophagus, the motility of the esophageal body must be carefully evaluated and, if inadequate, a partial fundoplication in conjunction with gastroplasty should be performed. Patients who have motility evidence of more than 50% interrupted or dropped contractions, or a history of several failed previous antireflux procedures, should be considered for esophageal resection.

Third, the surgeon should specifically question the patient for complaints of epigastric pain, nausea, vomiting, and loss of appetite. In the past, these symptoms were accepted as part of the reflux syndrome, but it is now known that they can be caused by excessive duodenogastric reflux, which occurs in approximately one third of patients with GERD.[2] This problem is most pronounced in patients who have had previous upper gastrointestinal surgery, particularly cholecystectomy, although this is not always the case.[25] In such patients, the correction of only the incompetent cardia may result in a disgruntled individual who continues to complain of nausea and epigastric pain on eating. In these patients, 24-hour pH monitoring of the stomach may help to detect and quantitate duodenogastric reflux.[26] The abnormality can also be documented with a ^{99m}Tc-HIDA scan when excessive reflux of radionuclide from the duodenum into the stomach can be demonstrated.[27] Antireflux surgery may reduce duodenogastric reflux by improving the efficiency of gastric emptying.[28] If surgery is necessary to control gastroesophageal reflux and if severe duodenogastric reflux is present, consideration should be given to performing a bile diversion procedure.[29]

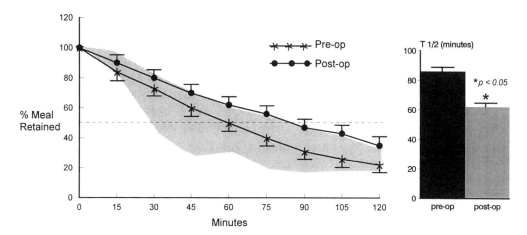

Fig. 3-5 Changes in gastric emptying of a semisolid meal following Nissen fundoplication. The shaded area represents the 10th and 90th percentiles of normal. (From Hinder RA, Stein HJ, Bremner CG, DeMeester TR. Relationship of a satisfactory outcome to normalization of delayed gastric emptying after a Nissen fundoplication. Ann Surg 210:458-465, 1989.)

Fourth, approximately 30% of patients with proved gastroesophageal reflux on 24-hour pH monitoring have hypersecretion on gastric analysis, and 2% to 3% of patients who have an antireflux operation will develop a gastric or duodenal ulcer.[30] These factors may modify the proposed antireflux procedure in patients with active ulcer disease or documentation of previous ulceration by the addition of a highly selective vagotomy.

Finally, delayed gastric emptying is found in approximately 40% of patients with GERD and can contribute to symptoms after an antireflux repair.[31] Usually, however, mild degrees of delayed gastric emptying are corrected by the antireflux procedure and there is a need for an additional gastric procedure only in patients with severe emptying disorders[28] (Fig. 3-5).

SELECTION OF SURGICAL APPROACH
Requirements for Antireflux Surgery

The requirements for antireflux surgery include (1) documentation of pathologic esophageal acid exposure on 24-hour pH monitoring, and (2) a mechanically defective LES.

If 24-hour esophageal pH monitoring is normal in a patient with unequivocal endoscopic esophagitis, the possibilities of alkaline, drug-induced, or retention esophagitis should be considered.[32] Patients with increased esophageal exposure to gastric juice in whom the sphincter is manometrically normal should be evaluated for a gastric or esophageal cause of reflux. Approximately 40% of these patients have gastric acid hypersecretion and respond to more aggressive antisecretory therapy. Patients with increased esophageal acid exposure, a mechanically defective sphincter, and no complications of the disease should be given the option of surgery as a cost-effective alternative.[12,33]

The goal of surgical treatment for GERD is to relieve the symptoms of reflux by the permanent restoration of cardioesophageal competence. This should be done without inducing dysphagia, which can occur when the outflow resistance of the reconstructed cardia exceeds the peristaltic power of the body of the esophagus. Achievement of this goal requires an understanding of the natural history of GERD, the status of the patient's esophageal function, and the selection of the appropriate antireflux procedure. We have based the selection of the surgical approach on body weight and an assessment of esophageal contractility and length. A transabdominal approach is used in nonobese patients with normal esophageal contractility and length. Obese patients or those with poor contractility or questionable esophageal length are approached transthoracically. Those with weak esophageal contractions and/or abnormal wave progression are treated with a partial fundoplication to avoid the increased outflow resistance associated with a complete fundoplication. If the esophagus is short after it is mobilized from diaphragm to aortic arch, a Collis gastroplasty is done to provide additional length and avoid placing the repair under tension. These patients are approached transthoracically and the length of the esophagus is again assessed after it is mobilized from the diaphragmatic hiatus to the aortic arch. The gastroesophageal junction is marked with a stitch, and if the length of the esophagus is insufficient to place a repair beneath the diaphragm without tension, the esophagus is considered to be short (Fig. 3-6).

In the majority of patients who have good esophageal contractility and normal

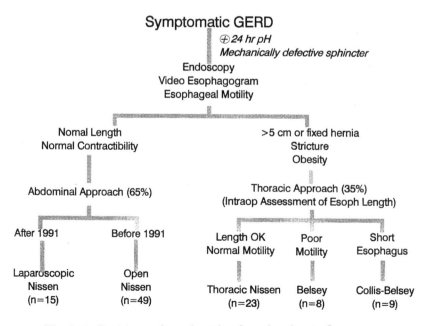

Fig. 3-6 Decision-making algorithm for tailored antireflux surgery.

esophageal length, the Nissen fundoplication is the procedure of choice for a primary antireflux repair. Experience and randomized studies have shown that the Nissen fundoplication is an effective and durable antireflux repair with minimal side effects while providing relief of reflux symptoms in 91% of patients for at least 10 years.[34] This is accomplished by restoring normal mechanical characteristics to a defective LES. Comparison of Nissen fundoplication to both symptomatic and continuous medical therapy in a recent Veterans Administration cooperative trial resulted in the conclusion that surgery was superior to medical therapy in every outcome measure used.[35] Furthermore, these results were consistent across the spectrum of institutions and surgical expertise encountered in this multi-institutional study, refuting arguments suggesting that antireflux surgery is only appropriate in the hands of esophageal specialists.[36]

RESULTS OF A TAILORED APPROACH

We have reviewed the outcome of such a selective approach in 104 patients with a wide spectrum of disease.[37] Our experience suggests that in approximately 65% of patients referred for surgery, a transabdominal Nissen fundoplication is the most suitable treatment. The remaining 35% of patients are best treated with an antireflux procedure tailored to the underlying abnormalities. Despite the presence of advanced disease in one third of the patients, this approach resulted in a clinical outcome similar to patients with early and less progressive disease (Table 3-1). Of interest, patients selected for a Belsey partial fundoplication because of poor motility in the presence of normal esophageal length benefited the least. This suggests that in patients with reflux disease a motility disorder in the presence of a normal esophageal length may be primary, rather than secondary, to the reflux disease.

The ideal therapy of GERD can be viewed conceptually along the continuum depicted in Fig. 3-7. The majority of patients requiring treatment have a relatively mild form of disease and respond to antisecretory medications. Patients with more severe forms of disease, particularly those with risk factors predictive of medical failure, or those who develop recurrent or progressive disease, should be considered for early definitive therapy. Laparoscopic Nissen fundoplication provides a long-

Table 3-1 Clinical outcome in 104 patients following a selective approach to antireflux surgery

Procedure	No. of Patients	Cured Patients	Failed Patients	% Cured
TAN/LN	49	44	5	90
TTN	20	19	1	95
Belsey	7	4	3	57
Collis-Belsey	9	8	1	88
	85	75	10	89

TAN/LN = transabdominal Nissen/laparoscopic Nissen; TTN = transthoracic Nissen.

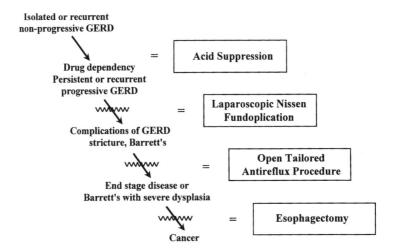

Fig. 3-7 Conceptual schema of the individual treatment at each stage of the spectrum of GERD.

term cure in the majority of these patients, with minimal discomfort, and an early return to normal activity. Patients who present with long-standing disease associated with poor esophageal function, a short esophagus, or stricture formation should undergo an open antireflux procedure tailored to their underlying anatomic and physiologic abnormalities. Finally, if the disease has progressed to frank esophageal failure, dysplastic Barrett's metaplasia, or esophageal adenocarcinoma, an esophagectomy will likely be required.

REFERENCES

1. Stein HJ, Eypasch EP, DeMeester TR, et al. Circadian esophageal motor function in patients with gastroesophageal reflux disease. Surgery 108:769-773, 1990.
2. Stein HJ, Barlow AP, DeMeester TR. Complications of gastroesophageal reflux disease: Role of the lower esophageal sphincter, esophageal acid and acid/alkaline exposure, and duodenogastric reflux. Ann Surg 216:35-43, 1992.
3. Vollan G, Stangeland L, Soreide JA, et al. Long term results after Nissen fundoplication and Belsey Mark IV operation in patients with reflux esophagitis and stricture. Eur J Surg 158:357-360, 1992.
4. Salama FD, Lamont G. Long-term results of the Belsey Mark IV antireflux operation in relation to the severity of esophagitis. J Thorac Cardiovasc Surg 100:517-519, 1990.
5. Little AG, Naunheim KS, Ferguson MK, et al. Surgical management of esophageal strictures. Ann Thorac Surg 45:144-147, 1988.
6. Luostarinen M, Isolauri J, Laitinen J, et al. Fate of Nissen fundoplication after 20 years. A clinical, endoscopical, and functional analysis. Gut 34:1015-1020, 1993.
7. Skinner DB, Belsey RHR. Surgical management of esophageal reflux and hiatus hernia. Long-term results with 1030 patients. J Thorac Cardiovasc Surg 53:33-54, 1967.
8. Zaninotto G, DeMeester TR, Schwizer W, et al. The lower esophageal sphincter in health and disease. Am J Surg 155:104-111, 1988.
9. Dent J. Australian clinical trials of omeprazole in the management of reflux oesophagitis. Digestion 47(Suppl):69-71, 1990.

10. Klinkenberg-Knol EC, Jansen JBMJ, Lamers CBHW, et al. Temporary cessation of long-term maintenance treatment with omeprazole in patients with H_2-receptor-antagonist-resistant reflux oesophagitis. Scand J Gastroenterol 25:1144-1150, 1990.

11. Lieberman DA. Medical therapy for chronic reflux esophagitis. Arch Intern Med 147:1717-1720, 1987.

12. Coley CM, Barry MJ, Spechler SJ, et al. Initial medical v. surgical therapy for complicated or chronic gastroesophageal reflux disease (GERD): A cost effective analysis. Gastroenterology 92:A138, 1993.

13. Ollyo JB, Monnier P, Fontolliet C, et al. The natural history and incidence of reflux oesophagitis. Gullet 3:3-10, 1993.

14. Ollyo JB, Lang F, Fontolliet CH, et al. Savary's new endoscopic grading of reflux-oesophagitis; A simple reproducible, logical, complete and useful classification. Gastroenterology 89:A100, 1990.

15. Hetzel DJ, Dent J, Reed WD, et al. Healing and relapse of severe peptic esophagitis after treatment with omeprazole. Gastroenterology 95:903, 1988.

16. Fontolliet C, Ollyo JB, Brossard E, et al. Barrett's esophagus may still progress. Gut 35(Suppl 4): A27, 1994.

17. Zaninotto G, DeMeester TR, Bremner CG, et al. Esophageal function in patients with reflux induced strictures and its relevance to surgical treatment. Ann Thorac Surg 47:362-370, 1989.

18. DeMeester TR. Barrett's esophagus. Surgery 113:239-240, 1993.

19. Stein JH, Hoeft S, DeMeester TR. Functional foregut abnormalities in Barrett's esophagus. J Thorac Cardiovasc Surg 105:107-111, 1993.

20. Sarr MG, Hamilton SR, Marone GC, et al. Barrett's esophagus: Its prevalence and association with adenocarcinoma in patients with symptoms of gastroesophageal reflux. Am J Surg 149:187-193, 1985.

21. DeMeester TR, Attwood SEA, Smyrk TC, et al. Surgical therapy in Barrett's esophagus. Ann Surg 212:528-542, 1990.

22. Altorki NK, Sanagawa M, Little AG, et al. High grade dysplasia in the columnar lined esophagus. Am J Surg 161:97-99, 1991.

23. Kahrilas PJ, Dodds WJ, Hogan WJ. Effect of peristaltic dysfunction on esophageal volume clearance. Gastroenterology 94:73-80, 1988.

24. Baue AE, Belsey RHR. The treatment of sliding hiatus hernia and reflux esophagitis by the Mark IV technique. Surgery 62:396, 1967.

25. Tolin RD, Malmud LS, Stelzer F, et al. Enterogastric reflux in normal subjects and patients with Billroth II gastroenterostomy: Measurement of enterogastric reflux. Gastroenterology 77:1027, 1979.

26. Fuchs KH, DeMeester TR, Hinder RA, et al. Computerized identification of pathologic duodenogastric reflux using 24-hour gastric pH monitoring. Ann Surg 213:13-20, 1991.

27. Stein HJ, Hinder RA, DeMeester TR, et al. Clinical use of 24-hour gastric pH monitoring vs. o-diisopropyl iminodiacetic acid (DISIDA) scanning in the diagnosis of pathologic duodenogastric reflux. Arch Surg 125:966-971, 1990.

28. Hinder RA, Stein HJ, Bremner CG, et al. Relationship of a satisfactory outcome to normalization of delayed gastric emptying after Nissen fundoplication. Ann Surg 210:458-465, 1989.

29. DeMeester TR, Fuchs KH, Ball CS, et al. Experimental and clinical results with proximal end-to-end duodenojejunostomy for pathologic duodenogastric reflux. Ann Surg 206:414-426, 1987.

30. Stein HJ, DeMeester T. Integrated ambulatory foregut monitoring in patients with functional foregut disorders. In Nyhus LM, ed. 1992 Surgery Annual, Part 1, vol. 24. Norwalk, Conn.: Appleton & Lange, 1992, pp 161-180.

31. Schwizer W, Hinder RA, DeMeester TR. Does delayed gastric emptying contribute to gastroesophageal reflux disease? Am J Surg 157:74, 1989.

32. Bonavina L, DeMeester TR, McChesney L, et al. Drug-induced esophageal strictures. Ann Surg 206:173-183, 1987.

33. Fuchs KH, DeMeester TR. Cost benefit aspects in the management of gastroesophageal reflux disease. In Siewert JR, Hölscher AH, eds. Diseases of the Esophagus. New York: Springer-Verlag, 1988, pp 857-861.

34. DeMeester TR, Bonavina L, Albertucci M. Nissen fundoplication for gastroesophageal reflux disease. Evaluation of primary repair in 100 consecutive patients. Ann Surg 204:9-20, 1986.
35. Spechler SJ, and the Department of Veterans Affairs Gastroesophageal Reflux Disease Study Group #277. Comparison of medical and surgical therapy for complicated gastroesophageal reflux disease in veterans. N Engl J Med 326:786-792, 1992.
36. Dunnington GL, DeMeester TR, and the Department of Veterans Affairs Gastroesophageal Reflux Disease Study Group. Outcome effect of adherence to operative principles of Nissen fundoplication by multiple surgeons. Am J Surg 166:654-658, 1993.
37. Kauer WKH, Peters JH, Ireland AP, et al. A tailored approach to antireflux surgery. J Cardiovasc Thorac Surg 109:1-7, 1995.

4

Barrett's Esophagus: Pathophysiology and Management

Geoffrey W.B. Clark, F.R.C.S.(Ed)

There has been an extraordinary increase in the incidence of esophageal adenocarcinoma in recent years[1,2] (Fig. 4-1). Barrett's esophagus is the only well-documented risk factor for the development of this cancer, which explains the renewed interest in this premalignant condition. Barrett's metaplasia is accepted to be the consequence of chronic gastroesophageal reflux disease (GERD), which links this common malady with one of the most lethal carcinomas. This chapter focuses on the new developments in understanding the pathophysiology of Barrett's esopha-

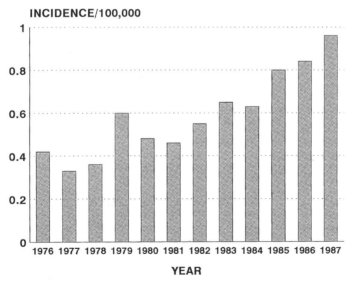

Fig. 4-1   The rising incidence of adenocarcinoma of the esophagus per 100,000 population in the United States reported by the SEER program for the years 1976 through 1987. (Personal communication: Dr. W. J. Blot, Biostatistics Branch, National Cancer Institute, NIH, Suite 431, Bethesda, MD 20892.)

gus, reviews the criteria for diagnosis, and addresses the controversies in management of benign and dysplastic Barrett's change.

PATHOPHYSIOLOGIC ABNORMALITIES

Patients with benign Barrett's esophagus have a combination of profound abnormalities in esophageal function.

Lower Esophageal Sphincter

More than 90% of patients with Barrett's esophagus have a mechanically defective lower esophageal sphincter (LES).[3-5] Manometrically, the LES has three components: (1) the resting sphincter pressure, (2) the overall length of the sphincter, and (3) the abdominal length. Normal values for each of these components in our laboratory are: resting pressure <6 mm Hg, overall length <2 cm, and abdominal length <1 cm.[6] Because resistance to flow is a function of pressure over length, sphincter incompetence is identified when any of the three components is below the normal limits. Resting sphincter pressures are lower in patients with Barrett's esophagus compared to both controls and patients with esophagitis[4] (Table 4-1). Patients with Barrett's esophagus tend to have reduced abdominal and overall sphincter lengths and often have multiple sphincter defects.[4]

Esophageal Body Motility

Esophageal body contractility is impaired in patients with Barrett's esophagus who have lower median contraction amplitudes in the distal esophagus[5] (Fig. 4-2) and an increased frequency of abnormal waveforms (dropped, interrupted, or simultaneous waves) compared to normal subjects. The impaired esophageal body motility results in poor clearance of refluxed material and allows prolonged contact times between the refluxing material and the esophageal mucosa with the production of a severe mucosal defect. Mason and Bremner[7] suggested that one factor re-

Table 4-1 Manometry of the lower esophageal sphincter*†

	Normals (n = 33)	Esophagitis (n = 31)	Barrett's (n = 22)
Resting pressure (mm Hg)	16.7 ± 1.0	8.7 ± 1.0‡	4.9 ± 0.8§
Overall length (cm)	4.2 ± 0.7	3.6 ± 0.6‡	3.2 ± 0.7‡
Abdominal length (cm)	2.6 ± 0.1	1.4 ± 0.1‡	1.1 ± 0.2‡

*Adapted from Iascone C, DeMeester TR, Little AG, et al. Barrett's esophagus. Functional assessment proposed pathogenesis and surgical therapy. Arch Surg 118:543-549, 1983.
†Values are expressed as mean and standard error of mean (SEM).
‡Indicates significant difference compared to normal subjects (p <0.05).
§Indicates a significant difference compared to patients with esophagitis.

sponsible for the length of the Barrett's segment was the severity of the esophageal body motor abnormality.

Acid Reflux

Most patients with Barrett's metaplasia have abnormal acid reflux into the distal esophagus,[3-5,8-10] which is best detected and quantified by 24-hour esophageal pH monitoring. Compared to patients with increased esophageal acid exposure but no columnar metaplasia, both the quality and quantity of the refluxate appear to be different in patients with Barrett's esophagus. Patients with Barrett's esophagus demonstrate an increased frequency and duration of reflux episodes compared to reflux patients with no columnar metaplasia.[4,11] There are reports of gastric hypersecretion associated with Barrett's esophagus with an elevated basal acid output compared to controls.[12-14] However, other investigators have not reproduced these findings.[15]

Alkaline Reflux

The observation that a columnar-lined esophagus can develop after total gastrectomy[16,17] indicates that reflux of acid is not a prerequisite for the development of Barrett's esophagus and suggests that irritation of the lower esophagus by the reflux of duodenal secretions (bile and pancreatic juice) may be as harmful as acid reflux. Attwood et al.[3] first reported an increased esophageal alkaline exposure in

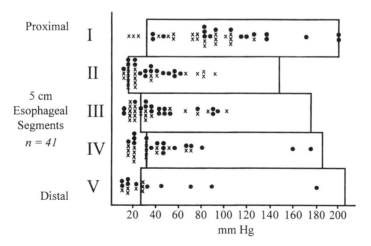

Fig. 4-2 Distribution of amplitude of esophageal contractions in 41 patients with Barrett's esophagus. The boxes represent the normal range (2.5th to 97.5th percentile) of amplitude for each 5 cm segment of the esophageal body. In patients with short esophagi, only three or four segments were able to be measured. • = uncomplicated Barrett's esophagus; x = complicated Barrett's esophagus. (From DeMeester TR, Attwood SEA, Smyrk TC, et al. Surgical therapy in Barrett's esophagus. Ann Surg 212:528-542, 1990.)

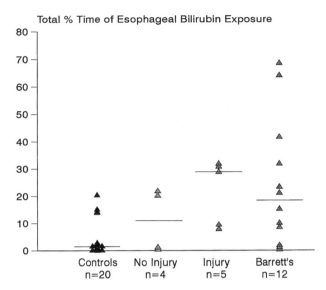

Fig. 4-3   Percentage of total study period during which the esophageal mucosa of each subject was exposed to bilirubin (i.e., absorbance >0.14). Values of each subject are plotted and the median of each group is denoted by the horizontal line. Patients with mucosal injury and Barrett's esophagus had a significantly higher bilirubin absorbance compared to controls (*p* <0.004, Mann-Whitney). (From Kauer WKH, Burdiles P, Ireland AP, et al. Does duodenal juice reflux into the esophagus of patients with complicated GERD? Evaluation of a fiberoptic sensor for bilirubin. Am J Surg 169:98-104, 1995.)

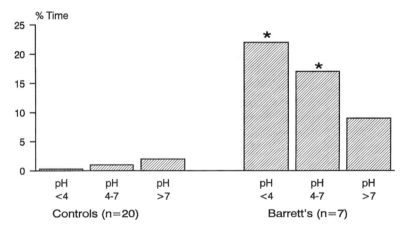

Fig. 4-4   Percentage of the time in the indicated pH intervals that the esophagus was exposed to bilirubin in controls and patients with Barrett's esophagus. Values are expressed as medians. * = Barrett's vs. controls (*p* <0.01 Mann-Whitney). (From Kauer WKH, Burdiles P, Ireland AP, et al. Does duodenal juice reflux into the esophagus of patients with complicated GERD? Evaluation of a fiberoptic sensor for bilirubin. Am J Surg 169:98-104, 1995.)

patients with Barrett's esophagus, based on observations made with 24-hour esophageal pH monitoring (measuring an increased time spent with the esophageal pH >7). This increased alkaline exposure was most pronounced in patients with complicated disease, those with stricture, ulceration, and dysplasia.[3] Some investigators have criticized the recording of esophageal pH >7 as a useful measurement[18] and have failed to identify elevated alkaline exposure in patients with complicated reflux disease.[19] However, prolonged esophageal aspiration studies[20-22] have supported the view that patients with Barrett's esophagus reflux have a complex mixture of acid and bile.

With the development of the "bile probe" by Bechi et al.,[23] a new tool has emerged that appears to be a more reliable method for the identification of bile reflux into the esophageal lumen. A fiberoptic cable is connected to a light source and data logger and is worn on the patient's belt (Bilitec 2000; Synectics Medical, Dallas, Tex.). The light source emits light at 453 nm, which is close to the maximum absorbance wavelength of bilirubin. The light is transmitted across a 2 mm space to a white Teflon reflector that reflects the light back to the probe. In the absence of bilirubin all the light emitted is reflected back, whereas in the presence of bilirubin the absorbance of light is directly related to the concentration of bilirubin, and the amount of light reflected back to the probe is proportionally reduced. The cable is passed through the nostril into the esophagus and positioned 5 cm above the upper border of the LES and the esophageal bilirubin exposure is monitored for 24 hours. With this technique it has been shown that patients with Barrett's esophagus have significantly higher levels of bile reflux into the lower esophagus compared to healthy controls[19,24] (Fig. 4-3). It is of interest to note that duodenal content has been repeatedly shown to promote the development of esophageal adenocarcinoma in rats.[25-27]

The term "alkaline reflux" has been used to describe reflux of duodenal content into the lower esophagus but may be a misnomer. Recent 24-hour studies with the combined esophageal bile probe and an esophageal pH electrode have indicated that bilirubin is frequently present in the esophageal lumen during episodes that register an acid pH on the pH electrode[24,28] (Fig. 4-4).

DIAGNOSIS

There is some controversy regarding the criteria for the diagnosis of Barrett's esophagus. Three histologic types of Barrett's epithelium have been described: (1) specialized "intestinal" type with villous architecture and goblet cells, (2) gastric fundic type with both chief and parietal cells, and (3) cardiac type with simple mucous glands but none of the other features. As there can be difficulty locating the exact site of the gastroesophageal junction at the time of endoscopy, and since the lower 2 cm of the esophagus may be lined by simple columnar epithelium in health, the 3 cm rule for Barrett's esophagus was established. This required that the abnormal-appearing mucosa extend at least 3 cm into the esophagus before Barrett's esophagus is diagnosed.

The rule is now being challenged based on the following observations:

1. Specialized intestinal-type epithelium is a premalignant metaplastic change, whereas identification of the junction- or fundic-type columnar metaplasia in the lower esophagus has considerably lower risk for malignant transformation, if these latter mucosal types are premalignant at all.

2. Endoscopic measurements of the location and length of columnar epithelium may be unreliable. In a multicenter controlled trial measurements of the length of Barrett's mucosa were not reproducible, even when performed by the same investigator only 6 weeks later.[29]

3. The presence of specialized metaplastic change at the gastroesophageal junction zone may not be apparent to the endoscopist. Such segments of cytologic change may be restricted to the area juxtaposed to the squamocolumnar junction and can only be diagnosed if biopsies are routinely taken from the gastroesophageal junction zone. Such biopsies are obtained with the retroflexed endoscope, although antegrade biopsies may also identify unsuspected Barrett's esophagus in this region. In a study of 87 patients with symptoms of GERD, biopsies from this location revealed five patients with unsuspected specialized intestinal metaplasia localized to the cardioesophageal junction zone, one of whom had high-grade dysplasia.[30] In none of the patients was the diagnosis of Barrett's esophagus suspected by the traditional antegrade examination, and the overall prevalence of Barrett's esophagus was increased from 18% to 24%. Zeroogian et al.[31] have reported similar findings of a high prevalence of short-segment Barrett's esophagus in patients in whom the gastroesophageal junction zone was routinely biopsied.

4. Short tongues of specialized intestinal metaplasia (<3 cm in length) may give rise to dysplastic change and adenocarcinoma.[32] In a study of 100 patients undergoing esophagogastrectomy for adenocarcinoma,[33] 42% of tumors located at the gastroesophageal junction were associated with specialized intestinal metaplasia. In most cases the Barrett's mucosa demonstrated dysplastic change, suggesting a Barrett's esophagus etiology. The length of Barrett's change associated with tumors at the gastroesophageal junction tended to be shorter (2.7 ± 1.8 cm) than that found associated with more proximal esophageal adenocarcinomas (7.3 ± 3.4 cm).

We investigated esophageal function in patients who had "short-segment" Barrett's mucosa, that is, specialized intestinal metaplasia measuring 3 cm or less on endoscopic examination. Fifty healthy volunteers, 29 patients with short-segment Barrett's esophagus, and 35 patients with extended Barrett's metaplasia were studied by esophageal manometry and 24-hour esophageal pH monitoring. Patients with short-segment Barrett's esophagus had a lower prevalence of a mechanically defective LES than patients with extended Barrett's esophagus (Fig. 4-5). Eighty-five percent of patients with short-segment Barrett's esophagus had increased esophageal acid exposure compared to 100% of those with extended Barrett's esophagus. Patients with short-segment disease had increased esophageal acid exposure compared to controls (Fig. 4-6), but spent less time at an acid pH than patients with more extensive Barrett's change. All lengths of Barrett's mucosa were

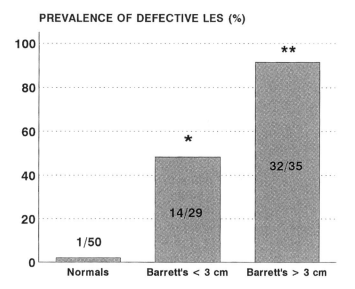

Fig. 4-5 Prevalence of a mechanically defective lower esophageal sphincter. * = p <0.01 vs. normals; ** = p <0.01 vs. normals and patients with short-segment Barrett's esophagus.

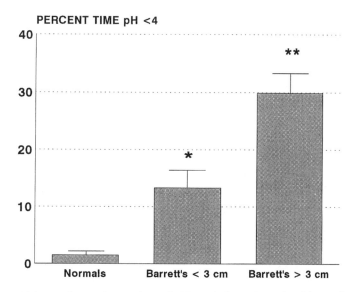

Fig. 4-6 Percent of the total time the esophageal pH was below 4 in each of the study groups. There was a significant difference between the groups (Kruscal Wallis, χ^2 = 82.8, 2 df, p <0.01). * = significant difference vs. normals (Mann-Whitney, p <0.01); ** = significant difference vs. normals and patients with short-segment Barrett's syndrome (Mann-Whitney, p <0.01).

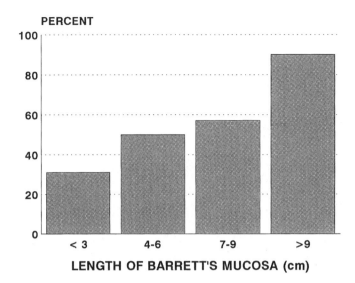

Fig. 4-7   Prevalence of complications and length of Barrett's mucosa. Longer lengths of Barrett's esophagus were more commonly associated with complications ($\chi^2 = 10.9$, 3 df, $p < 0.01$).

associated with a profound reduction in the contraction amplitudes in the distal esophagus. Complications (stricture, ulcer, and dysplasia) were more commonly associated with longer lengths of Barrett's change (Fig. 4-7). However, patients with short-segment Barrett's mucosa must be considered to have a premalignant condition because 17% had dysplasia.

Short-segment Barrett's esophagus appears to be commonly associated with GERD. The presence of a competent LES may restrict the extent of the metaplastic process to the gastroesophageal junction. Short segments of specialized intestinal metaplasia appear to be premalignant in nature. It is proposed that the 3 cm rule represents a restrictive definition of Barrett's esophagus. The identification of specialized intestinal mucosa in any biopsy is sufficient grounds for making a diagnosis of Barrett's esophagus independent of the extent of the endoscopically observed abnormalities. Such a diagnosis carries with it a premalignant potential and the need for surveillance.

PREMALIGNANT POTENTIAL

Barrett's esophagus is a premalignant lesion. Patients are at an increased risk of developing adenocarcinoma that is between 30 and 125 times higher than that of the normal population. Figures estimating the risk of malignancy in patients with Barrett's esophagus are best established by prospective studies. Hameeteman et al.[34] cited the highest risk with 5 of 50 patients followed up for a mean duration of 5.2 years developing esophageal adenocarcinoma. That is equivalent to an incidence of

Table 4-2 The risk of benign Barrett's esophagus progressing to adenocarcinoma

Authors	No. of Cases	Mean Duration of Follow-Up (years)	No. of Cases of Esophageal Adenocarcinoma	Incidence (patient years)	Risk
Hameeteman et al.[34]	50	5.2	5	1:52	×125
Robertson et al.[35]	56	2.8	3	1:56	×62
Sprung et al.[36]	41	NS	2	1:81	—
Spechler et al.[37]	105	3.3	2	1:175	×40
VanDerVeen et al.[38]	155	4.4	4	1:170	×30
Cameron et al.[39]	104	8.5	2	1:441	×30
Iftikhar et al.[40]	102	4.4	4	1:115	×30

NS = not significant.

1 in 52 patient years of follow-up. Several prospective studies reported the risk of developing esophageal adenocarcinoma in patients with Barrett's esophagus (Table 4-2).

ENDOSCOPIC SURVEILLANCE

Patients with Barrett's esophagus are at an increased risk for the development of esophageal adenocarcinoma that is 30 to 125 times that of the normal population and, expressed as adenocarcinomas per 100,000 patients with Barrett's esophagus per year, is on the magnitude 500 per 100,000 cases. It is currently recommended for patients with Barrett's esophagus who are medically fit to be enrolled in a surveillance program and undergo annual endoscopy examination with multiple biopsies. An acceptable protocol for these purposes requires four biopsies, one from each quadrant of the esophagus, and for every 2 cm along the visible length of the Barrett's mucosa, with additional biopsies from any abnormal-appearing area. Patients with low-grade dysplasia should be screened at 6-month intervals. If high-grade dysplasia is confirmed by two experienced pathologists, esophageal resection should be considered unless the patient is medically unfit. In that case continued surveillance is undertaken every 3 months until adenocarcinoma is diagnosed.

MANAGEMENT
Barrett's Esophagus Free of Dysplasia

The diagnosis of Barrett's esophagus is usually made during investigation of patients with symptoms of GERD. The majority will initially be treated with medical therapy using H_2 receptor blockers or the proton pump–inhibitor omeprazole. Despite the widespread and liberal prescribing of these powerful acid-suppressing drugs, there continues to be a substantial number of patients with Barrett's esophagus resistant to medical therapy. The major reason is because medical therapy does not address the underlying problem, which is a mechanically defective LES, and the regurgitation of gastric juice continues unabated. Because drug therapy is focused on acid suppression, a potential problem is the continued reflux of alkaline material (duodenal juice containing bile and pancreatic enzymes). As already mentioned, increased esophageal alkaline exposure is associated with complications in Barrett's esophagus, including stricture, ulcer, and dysplasia, and may explain why 10% to 20% of patients with GERD fail to heal mucosal injury despite profound acid suppression.[41,42]

Criteria for an antireflux operation in patients with uncomplicated Barrett's esophagus are a mechanically defective LES on stationary manometry and increased esophageal acid exposure on 24-hour esophageal pH monitoring. An antireflux procedure is preferred in patients with Barrett's esophagus since the operation corrects the mechanical problem, restores LES function, and abolishes reflux of all gastric and duodenal content into the esophagus, thereby preventing repetitive injury to the Barrett's mucosa and the normal esophageal mucosa.[5] An antireflux procedure is superior to medical therapy in the management of complicated reflux disease.[43] Further, Nissen fundoplication is the only therapy that has been shown to be effective in the long-term control of reflux disease.[44]

It seems prudent for patients with Barrett's esophagus to remain in an endoscopic surveillance program following antireflux surgery since there is no reliable evidence to indicate that the Barrett's mucosa will regress. However, the important question is whether the antireflux procedure can prevent progression of the Barrett's mucosa. There are several reports of adenocarcinoma developing in Barrett's esophagus after antireflux operations but none included efforts to exclude dysplasia before surgery or to document the effectiveness of the repair after surgery. Whether a properly functioning antireflux repair can indeed reduce the rate of malignant progression in Barrett's esophagus awaits confirmation. One prospective registry showed that medical therapy was associated with a significantly higher incidence of dysplasia and adenocarcinoma than surgical therapy.[45]

Barrett's Esophagus With Low-Grade Dysplasia

Patients who are diagnosed as indefinite for dysplasia or as low-grade dysplasia should undergo a repeat endoscopic examination with meticulous examination of the Barrett's epithelium and documentation of the location of any areas of mucosal irregularity. Biopsies should be obtained along the length of the mucosa in the standard fashion and the location of each biopsy should be recorded. Following examination of the histologic specimens, the presence and extent of the dysplastic change can be documented. Because inflammatory atypia can be confused with low-grade dysplasia, patients who have not been treated for their reflux disease should receive a 3-month course of intensive acid suppression with omeprazole, 20 to 40 mg daily, to reduce the active inflammation. After this course of treatment, endoscopy should be repeated and the esophagus should be extensively biopsied, paying particular attention to areas previously reported to show dysplastic change. If the low-grade dysplasia persists, the patient should undergo an antireflux procedure followed by endoscopic surveillance with multiple biopsies every 6 months.

Barrett's Esophagus With High-Grade Dysplasia

High-grade dysplasia is a sinister finding. It is presently the best available marker of patients with Barrett's esophagus who will develop adenocarcinoma or who are already harboring an invasive carcinoma. An aggressive approach to these patients is recommended. Experienced surgeons have been struck by the difficulty in the differentiation of high-grade dysplasia from adenocarcinoma on the basis of endoscopic biopsy examination. Several studies[46-49] have indicated that up to 50% of patients who undergo esophagectomy for high-grade dysplasia already have invasive adenocarcinoma. In our experience of nine patients who were operated on with a diagnosis of high-grade dysplasia, five (55%) had unexpected invasive adenocarcinoma in the resected specimen.[50] Despite obtaining a considerable number of preoperative biopsies, the presence of invasive adenocarcinoma was frequently missed. Patients with mucosal abnormalities were more likely to have adenocarcinoma, but a normal-appearing Barrett's mucosa did not indicate the absence of underlying adenocarcinoma.

Some authors have preferred a conservative approach to the management of high-grade dysplasia because surgical therapy has been considered to have a high morbidity and, in a few cases, mortality has occurred in patients who were free from invasive cancer in the resected specimen.[51-53] Fundamental to this hypothesis is the ability to distinguish high-grade dysplasia from early adenocarcinoma by endoscopic biopsy. Other concerns with continued surveillance for high-grade dysplasia are that the majority of patients will progress to adenocarcinoma within a relatively short period of time, thereby negating the rationale for continuing surveillance.

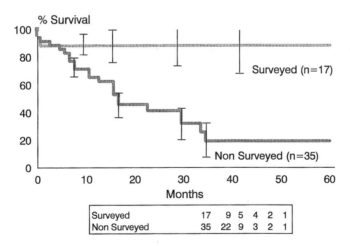

Fig. 4-8 Survival after esophageal resection in endoscopically surveyed and nonsurveyed patients. There was a significant difference between the groups (log rank $\chi^2 = 5.8$, $p < 0.05$). Bars indicate standard errors of the mean. Surveyed group included 13 patients with adenocarcinoma and four with high-grade dysplasia. The number of patients at each year of follow-up are shown in the key box. (From Peters JH, Clark GWB, Ireland AP, et al. Outcome of adenocarcinoma arising in Barrett's esophagus in endoscopically surveyed and nonsurveyed patients. J Thorac Cardiovasc Surg 108:813-822, 1994.)

Hameeteman et al.,[34] in a prospective study, reported on five patients with Barrett's adenocarcinoma who progressed from low-grade to high-grade dysplasia prior to the development of cancer. The time interval from low-grade dysplasia to carcinoma was only 1.5 to 4 years. High-grade dysplasia is considered to be a marker for early esophageal adenocarcinoma and patients who are medically fit should undergo esophagectomy with anticipation of permanent cure of the disease. Continued surveillance should be reserved for older patients and those with coexisting medical conditions in whom resection would only be undertaken if adenocarcinoma develops.

Endoscopic surveillance for patients with Barrett's esophagus followed by early surgical resection for high-grade dysplasia or intramucosal adenocarcinoma is an effective management policy since such patients have an improved outcome compared to patients with newly recognized Barrett's carcinomas who were not under surveillance. Esophageal resection was performed in 52 patients for either high-grade dysplasia or adenocarcinoma arising in Barrett's esophagus.[50] The patients were divided into two groups: (1) 17 patients who had been referred for surgical consultation after a diagnosis of high-grade dysplasia or adenocarcinoma had been made during endoscopic surveillance; and (2) 35 patients who were not part of an endoscopic surveillance program and who developed a de novo adenocarcinoma. A significant survival advantage was obtained in those patients in the surveyed group compared to nonsurveyed patients (Fig. 4-8).

REFERENCES

1. Blot WJ, Devesa SS, Kneller RW, et al. Rising incidence of adenocarcinoma of the esophagus and gastric cardia. JAMA 265:1287-1289, 1991.
2. Hesketh PJ, Clapp RW, Doos WG, et al. The increasing frequency of adenocarcinoma of the esophagus. Cancer 64:526-530, 1989.
3. Attwood SEA, DeMeester TR, Bremner CG, et al. Alkaline gastroesophageal reflux: Implications in the development of complications in Barrett's columnar-lined lower esophagus. Surgery 106: 764-770, 1989.
4. Iascone C, DeMeester TR, Little AG, et al. Barrett's esophagus. Functional assessment, proposed pathogenesis and surgical therapy. Arch Surg 118:543-549, 1983.
5. DeMeester TR, Attwood SEA, Smyrk TC, et al. Surgical therapy in Barrett's esophagus. Ann Surg 212:528-542, 1990.
6. Zaninotto G, DeMeester TR, Schwizer W. The lower esophageal sphincter in health and disease. Am J Surg 155:104-110, 1988.
7. Mason RJ, Bremner CG. Motility differences between long-segment and short-segment Barrett's esophagus. Am J Surg 165:686-689, 1993.
8. Skinner DB, Walther BC, Riddell RH, et al. Barrett's esophagus—Comparison of benign and malignant cases. Ann Surg 198:554-566, 1983.
9. Stein HJ, Barlow AP, DeMeester TR, et al. Complications of gastroesophageal reflux disease. The role of the lower esophageal sphincter, esophageal acid/alkaline exposure, and duodenogastric reflux. Ann Surg 216:35-43, 1992.
10. Winters C Jr, Spurling TJ, Chobanian SJ, et al. Barrett's esophagus. A prevalent, occult complication of gastroesophageal reflux disease. Gastroenterology 92:118-124, 1987.
11. Gillen P, Keeling P, Bryne PJ, et al. Barrett's oesophagus: pH profile. Br J Surg 74:774-776, 1987.

12. Collen MJ, Lewis JH, Benjamin SB. Gastric acid hypersecretion in refractory gastroesophageal reflux disease. Gastroenterology 98:654-661, 1990.

13. Collen MJ, Johnson DA. Correlation between basal acid output and daily ranitidine dose required for therapy in Barrett's esophagus. Dig Dis Sci 37:570-576, 1992.

14. Mulholland MW, Reid BJ, Levine DS, et al. Elevated gastric acid secretion in patients with Barrett's metaplastic epithelium. Dig Dis Sci 34:1329-1335, 1989.

15. Hirschowitz BI. A critical analysis with appropriate controls of gastric acid and pepsin secretion in clinical esophagitis. Gastroenterology 101:1149-1158, 1991.

16. Meyer W, Vollmar F, Bar W. Barrett's esophagus following total gastrectomy. A contribution to its pathogenesis. Endoscopy 2:121-126, 1979.

17. Morrow D, Passaro ER Jr. Alkaline reflux esophagitis after total gastrectomy. Am J Surg 132:287-291, 1976.

18. Singh S, Bradley LA, Richter JE. Determinants of esophageal "alkaline" pH environment in controls and patients with gastroesophageal reflux disease. Gut 34:309-316, 1993.

19. Champion G, Singh S, Bechi P, et al. Duodenogastric reflux—Relationship to esophageal pH and response to omeprazole. Gastroenterology (Suppl) 104:A51, 1993.

20. Gotley DC, Morgan AP, Cooper MJ. Bile acid concentrations in the refluxate of patients with reflux oesophagitis. Br J Surg 75:587-590, 1988.

21. Iftikar SY, Ledingham S, Steele RJC, et al. Bile reflux in the columnar-lined oesophagus. Ann R Coll Surg Engl 75:411-416, 1993.

22. Stein HJ, Feussner H, Kauer W, et al. "Alkaline" gastroesophageal reflux: Assessment by ambulatory esophageal aspiration and pH monitoring. Am J Surg 167:163-168, 1994.

23. Bechi P, Pucciani F, Baldini F, et al. Long-term ambulatory enterogastric reflux monitoring. Validation of a new fiberoptic technique. Dig Dis Sci 38:1297-1306, 1993.

24. Kauer WKH, Burdiles P, Ireland AP, et al. Does duodenal juice reflux into the esophagus of patients with complicated GERD? Evaluation of a fiberoptic sensor for bilirubin. Am J Surg 169:98-104, 1995.

25. Pera M, Cardesa A, Bombi JA, et al. Influence of esophagoduodenostomy on the induction of adenocarcinoma of the distal esophagus in Sprague-Dawley rats by the subcutaneous injection of 2,6 dimethylnitrosomorpholine. Cancer Res 49:6803-6808, 1989.

26. Attwood SEA, Smyrk TC, DeMeester TR, et al. Duodenoesophageal reflux and the development of esophageal adenocarcinoma in the rats. Surgery 111:503-510, 1992.

27. Clark GWB, Smyrk TC, Mirvish SS, et al. The effect of gastroduodenal juice and dietary fat on the development of Barrett's esophagus and esophageal neoplasia: An experimental rat model. Ann Surg Oncol 1:252-261, 1994.

28. Kauer WKH, Ireland AP, Burdiles P, et al. The correlation between bile and acid reflux in Barrett's esophagus. Gastroenterology 106:A104, 1994.

29. Kim SL, Waring P, Spechler SJ, et al. Diagnostic inconsistencies in Barrett's esophagus. Gastroenterology 107:945-949, 1994.

30. Clark GWB, Ireland AP, Chandrasoma P, et al. Inflammation and metaplasia in the transitional epithelium of the gastroesophageal junction: A new marker for gastroesophageal reflux disease. Gastroenterology 106:A63, 1994.

31. Zeroogian JM, Spechler SJ, Antonioli DA, et al. The high incidence of short segment Barrett's esophagus. Gastroenterology 106:A216, 1994.

32. Schnell TG, Sontag SJ, Chejfec G. Adenocarcinomas arising in tongues or short segments of Barrett's esophagus. Dig Dis Sci 37:137-143, 1992.

33. Clark GWB, Smyrk TC, Burdiles P, et al. Is Barrett's metaplasia the source of adenocarcinomas of the cardia? Arch Surg 129:609-614, 1994.

34. Hameeteman W, Tytgat GNJ, Houthoff HJ, et al. Barrett's esophagus: Development of dysplasia and adenocarcinoma. Gastroenterology 96:1249-1256, 1989.

35. Robertson CS, Mayberry JF, Nicholson DA, et al. Value of endoscopic surveillance in the detection of neoplastic change in Barrett's oesophagus. Br J Surg 75:760-763, 1988.

36. Sprung DJ, Ellis FH, Cibb SP. Incidence of adenocarcinoma in Barrett's esophagus [abstract]. Am J Gastroenterol 79:817, 1984.
37. Spechler SJ, Robbins AH, Bloomfield Rubins H, et al. Adenocarcinoma and Barrett's esophagus: An overrated risk? Gastroenterology 87:927-933, 1984.
38. VanDerVeen AH, Dees J, Blankenstein JD, et al. Adenocarcinoma in Barrett's oesophagus; An overrated risk. Gut 30:14-18, 1989.
39. Cameron AJ, Ott BJ, Payne WS. The incidence of adenocarcinoma in columnar-lined (Barrett's) esophagus. N Engl J Med 313:857-859, 1985.
40. Iftikhar SY, James PD, Steele RJC, et al. Length of Barrett's oesophagus: An important factor in the development of dysplasia and adenocarcinoma. Gut 33:1155-1158, 1992.
41. Hetzel DJ, Dent J, Reed WD, et al. Healing and relapse of severe peptic esophagitis after treatment with omeprazole. Gastroenterology 95:903-912, 1988.
42. Klinkenberg-Knol EC, Jansen JMBJ, Festen HPM, et al. Double-blind multicenter comparison of omeprazole and ranitidine in the treatment of reflux esophagitis. Lancet 1:349-351, 1987.
43. Spechler SJ, and the Department of Veterans Affairs Gastroesophageal Reflux Disease Study Group #277. Comparison of medical and surgical therapy for complicated gastroesophageal reflux disease in veterans. N Engl J Med 326:786-792, 1992.
44. DeMeester TR, Bonavina L, Albertucci M. Nissen fundoplication for gastroesophageal reflux disease; Evaluation of primary repair in 100 consecutive patients. Ann Surg 204:9-20, 1986.
45. McCallum RW, Polepalle S, Davenport K, et al. Role of anti-reflux surgery against dysplasia in Barrett's esophagus. Gastroenterology 100:A121, 1991.
46. Pera M, Trastek VF, Carpenter HA, et al. Barrett's esophagus with high grade dysplasia an indication for esophagectomy? Ann Thorac Surg 54:199-204, 1992.
47. Altorki NK, Sanagawa M, Little AG, et al. High grade dysplasia in the columnar lined esophagus. Am J Surg 161:97-99, 1991.
48. Rice TW, Falk GW, Achkar E, et al. Surgical management of high grade dysplasia in Barrett's esophagus. Am J Gastroenterol 88:1832-1836, 1993.
49. Streitz JM, Andrews CW, Ellis FH. Endoscopic surveillance of Barrett's esophagus. Does it help? J Thorac Cardiovasc Surg 105:383-388, 1993.
50. Peters JH, Clark GWB, Ireland AP, et al. Outcome of adenocarcinoma arising in Barrett's esophagus in endoscopically surveyed and nonsurveyed patients. J Thorac Cardiovasc Surg 108:813-822, 1994.
51. Levine DS, Haggitt RC, Blount PL, et al. An endoscopic biopsy protocol can differentiate high grade dysplasia from early adenocarcinoma in Barrett's esophagus. Gastroenterology 105:40-50, 1993.
52. Cameron AJ, Carpenter HC, Trastek VF. Barrett's esophagus with high grade dysplasia: Is resection required? Gastroenterology 106:A375, 1994.
53. Reid BJ, Weinstein WM, Lewin KJ, et al. Endoscopic biopsy can detect high grade dysplasia or early adenocarcinoma in Barrett's esophagus without grossly recognizable neoplastic lesions. Gastroenterology 94:81-90, 1988.

5

Laparoscopic Approach to Gastroesophageal Reflux Disease

Marco Anselmino, M.D. • *Giovanni Zaninotto, M.D.*
Ermanno Ancona, M.D.

Video-assisted laparoscopic surgery has changed the approach to many problems in general surgery and the encouraging results obtained with laparoscopic cholecystectomy and appendectomy have led many surgeons to apply minimally invasive access to more surgical procedures. Results comparable with those of the corresponding open techniques, but with less surgical trauma, shorter hospitalization, lower morbidity, and a shorter convalescence, have been obtained after laparoscopic removal of common bile duct stones,[1] repair of groin hernias,[2] large and small bowel resection,[3,4] and myotomy of the esophagus.[5] Among the new surgical procedures, laparoscopic antireflux surgery has gained widespread popularity since its first report in 1991[6] and is no longer in the experimental phase.

Gastroesophageal reflux symptoms are very common, but abnormal esophageal acid exposure as assessed by 24-hour pH monitoring[7] is only found in 65% of symptomatic cases. Of these patients 50% to 60% have a manometrically defective lower esophageal sphincter (LES)[8] and form a subset that benefits from surgical treatment.[9,10] Unfortunately, many surgeons now practicing laparoscopic antireflux surgery lack previous experience with the corresponding open type of antireflux surgery. Approach and mobilization of the intra-abdominal esophagus are feasible laparoscopically in the absence of previous abdominal surgery and excessive esophageal shortening.[6,11] Large hiatal or paraesophageal hernias can be reduced into the abdomen by expert hands using "dedicated" instruments. A high degree of hands-on skills, confidence with laparoscopic imaging, and specific surgical supplies are needed during the laparoscopic hiatus preparation and fundoplication, making this advanced laparoscopic surgery. When the indications for surgical treatment are correct and the surgical steps of conventional operations are fully respected, laparoscopic correction of gastroesophageal reflux produces results comparable with those of the corresponding open procedure. A good knowledge of the pathophysiology of gastroesophageal reflux disease (GERD), additional skills beyond those acquired in performing laparoscopic cholecystectomy, and experience with all aspects of open antireflux surgery are consequently essential.

GENERAL PRINCIPLES OF ANTIREFLUX SURGERY AND PATIENT SELECTION FOR LAPAROSCOPIC TREATMENT

As in the case of open surgery, the indication for laparoscopic antireflux repair remains a documented abnormal exposure of the distal esophagus to gastric acid, with or without hiatal hernia, which occurs more often in patients with a defective LES.[8] Patients usually have a history of at least 6 months of medical, dietary, and postural therapy. Surgery is required if symptoms recur when the treatment is stopped or if symptoms and esophagitis fail to respond to acid suppressants. Diagnostic workup includes endoscopy with multiple biopsies, barium swallow, esophageal manometry, and 24-hour pH monitoring. In selected cases, gastric emptying studies are also useful. Endoscopy evaluates mucosal damage of the distal esophagus and, in association with esophagography, provides information on the presence and type of hiatal hernia and on any complications, such as peptic stricture. Stationary manometry measures the resting tone and length of the LES and the degree of esophageal motor dysfunction. Together with 24-hour pH monitoring of the distal esophagus, manometric study enables a functional evaluation of the disease and establishes the indication for surgery.

The aim of laparoscopic antireflux repair is to reduce any hiatal hernia and treat the reflux problem by restoring cardia competency, increasing its mechanical function, and allowing for normal swallowing, belching, and vomiting. These goals are also achieved via the laparoscopic approach by creating a plication around the distal esophagus after repositioning an adequate length of distal esophagus into the abdomen.[10] On the basis of experience with open antireflux surgery, the laparoscopic fundoplication constructed using the gastric fundus, hepatic round ligament (teres ligament), or prosthetic silicon materials has recently been proposed.[6,12-16] Since the operation should enable the new sphincter to relax, the best tissue to use for an antireflux plication is the gastric fundus, which is able to relax synchronously with the LES in response to deglutition.[17] To prevent postoperative dysphagia, the plication should not increase the new sphincter's resistance during relaxation, which could overcome the strength of the peristaltic contractions and cause food impaction. Sphincter resistance is determined by the length, shape, and caliber of the plication. A 2 cm long total (or partial in the case of defective peristalsis) gastric fundoplication, fashioned around a 50 to 60 F dilator inserted in the esophagus, is the recommended technique.[9,14] Surgical correction must also guarantee that the new sphincter is kept inside the abdomen without tension. Closure of the diaphragmatic crura with one to three sutures usually prevents the fundoplication from slipping into the chest (Fig. 5-1). When there is too much tension, or the esophagus is short, it is worth considering making the esophagus longer (such as the Collis gastroplasty) and converting the operation to an open procedure. Conversion to laparotomy must not be considered as a failure and the laparoscopic surgeon must avoid the temptation to simplify well-established techniques to expedite laparoscopic completion. Uncontrollable bleeding and esophageal or gastric perforation are the most common indications for conversion. Difficulty in taking down the short gastric vessels, inadequate proximal gastric mobilization, or difficulty in repositioning the esophagogastric junction below the hiatus add the risk of wrap-

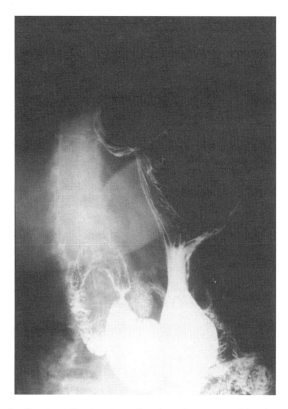

Fig. 5-1   Nissen fundoplication slipping into the chest in a case of inadequate closure of the diaphragmatic crura.

ping the stomach instead of the esophagus and should prompt the laparoscopic surgeon to convert to laparotomy. The laparoscopic surgeon must avoid the creation of tight wraps, which increase the likelihood of postoperative dysphagia or gas bloat and the recurrence of symptoms caused by fundoplication dysfunction.

The total posterior gastric fundoplication (Nissen) is currently the most-performed laparoscopic antireflux procedure[6,13,14] (Table 5-1). Laparoscopic 270-degree posterior (Toupet) and anterior (Dor) gastric hemifundoplications have proved effective in patients with GERD complicated by poor esophageal body function[14] and in patients with achalasia after extramucosal Heller's myotomy has been performed.[5] The laparoscopic placement of the Angelchick silicon prosthesis[16] or the creation of an antireflux mechanism using the hepatic round ligament instead of the gastric fundus[15] are also used to control abnormal gastroesophageal reflux.

EQUIPMENT

The imaging system used in laparoscopic antireflux procedures consists of a 10 mm 0-degree laparoscope. A 10 mm 30-degree optic can be used when vision of the left and right lateral aspects of the intra-abdominal esophagus must be improved to

Table 5-1 Results of various laparoscopic antireflux procedures

Author	Year	No. of Patients	Technique	Conversion (%)	Follow-up (months)	Good Results (%)	Transient Dysphagia (%)	Persistent Dysphagia* (%)	Recurrent Reflux (%)
Dallemagne et al.[6]	1991 p	12	Nissen	25	1	77	0	—	—
Bagnato[18]	1992 p	14	Nissen	14	—	100	0	—	—
Weerts et al.[19]	1993 p	132	Nissen	3	>3	93	5	2	1
Cuschieri[20]	1993 p	18	Lig. teres cardiopexy (n = 9); Nissen (n = 4); Toupet (n = 5)	0	3	100	—	—	0
Mutter et al.[21]	1993 p	10	Nissen-Rossetti	0	6	90	10	—	0
MacPhee[22]	1993 p	11	Angelchick	0	34	91	0	—	9
Hinder et al.[14]	1994 p	198	Nissen (with pledgets)	3	6-32	92	25	6	1
Cadiere et al.[23]	1994 p	80	Nissen	4	1-12	92	1	0	0
Collard et al.[12]	1994 p	39	Nissen (n = 33); Toupet (n = 2); Lortat-Jacob (n = 2)	5	11	88	3	—	5
Jamieson et al.[24]	1994 p	155	Nissen	12	9	98	5	—	0
Bittner et al.[25]	1994 p	35	Nissen (with pledgets)	14	3-6	87	24	—	—
Materia et al.[26]	1994 a	62	Nissen	0	5.2	97	16	3	—
DelGenio et al.[27]	1994 a	22	Nissen	0	9-19	93	6	7	0
Cady[28]	1994 a	150	(agraffes) (n = 135); (stistches) (n = 13)	1	>18	95	—	3	2
Hallerback et al.[29,30]	1994 a-p	60	Nissen-Rossetti	15	3-8	97	0	0	—
Feussner and Stein[31]	1994 p	18	Nissen-Rossetti	17	—	100	11	8	0
Boulez et al.[32]	1994 a	117	Nissen-Rossetti	0	—	86	—	2	3
Fingerhut et al.[33]	1994 a	148	Nissen	7	3.5	92	11	—	—
Peracchia et al.[34]	1994 p	25	Nissen-Rossetti	4	2-25	95	8	—	0
Ancona et al.[35]	1994 p	24	Nissen-Rossetti (n = 19); Toupet (n = 2)	12	1-25	91	14	9	0
Ancona et al.[36]	1994 p	183	Nissen (n = 35); Nissen-Rossetti (n = 137); Dor (n = 10); Toupet (n = 1)	5	—	95	9	4	1
		1513		5.4		92.8	8.2	4.0	1.4

p = publication; a = abstract.
*Requiring reoperation or dilation.

complete dissection from the diaphragmatic crura. Under general anesthesia and with the patient in the lithotomy reversed Trendelenburg position, pneumoperitoneum is established at 10 to 12 mm Hg using a Veress needle or open Hasson technique. Five trocars are required, but their positioning varies according to which technique is being used. Fig. 5-2 illustrates the trocar sites during the laparoscopic Nissen and Toupet techniques. The laparoscope is inserted through a 10 mm trocar positioned in the midline, three to four finger breadths above the umbilicus (No. 1). A second 10 mm trocar, inserted on the right side just above the midpoint of the hemitransverse umbilical line, is for the three finger breadths liver retractor (No. 2). A 5 mm trocar, positioned on the left side at the same level as the second trocar, but more laterally on the anterior axillary line, is for a clamp that pulls down the stomach during esophageal dissection and proximal gastric preparation (No. 3). Two other trocars, one 5 mm and one 10 mm, represent the two operative ports. The first is introduced just below the xiphoid, 1 cm to the right of the midline (No. 4), and the second is inserted at the same level as the No. 3 trocar in the midpoint between the No. 3 and No. 1 trocars (No. 5). All laparoscopic antireflux techniques use both standard and specifically designed instruments. Atraumatic forceps and clamps ensure manipulation, whereas dissection is performed using graspers, hooks, or scissors with electrocautery. Some of these instruments have a finger-controlled shaft rotation that permits turning of the distal tip without abnormal twisting of the wrist. A new reticulator version of graspers permits articulation of the instrument's distal tip to an angle greater than 90 degrees and is useful during fundoplication because it facilitates the passage of the gastric fundus through the window created behind the dissected esophagus.

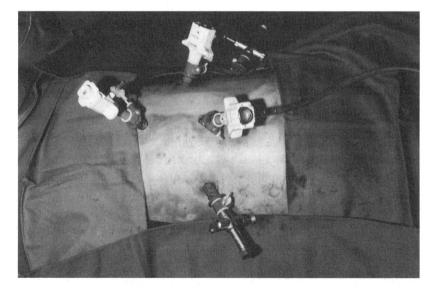

Fig. 5-2   Position of trocars during laparoscopic Nissen and Toupet procedures.

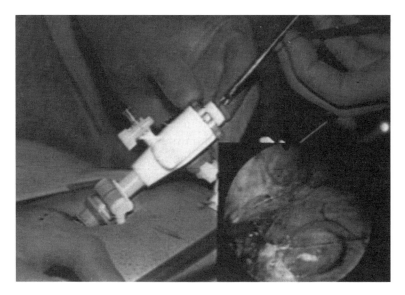

Fig. 5-3 Extracorporeal knot tying uses monofilament sutures by fashioning a hemikey introduced into the abdomen by a special knot pusher. To guarantee effective tying, five to six knots are necessary.

An efficient high-flow irrigator/aspirator unit is required to control bleeding and preserve a clean operative field. Short gastric vessels or other possible sources of bleeding can easily be clipped using Endo Clip applicators. Intracorporeal suturing and knot tying are among the advanced operative skills that laparoscopic surgeons must master. Standard or specifically designed needle holders are used, and nonabsorbable suture materials with short and straight needles are specifically customized. Wrap fixation can be simplified, however, by an extracorporeal knot-tying technique that uses a special knot pusher (Fig. 5-3), or by using agraffes stapled between the two limbs of the fundoplication.

TECHNIQUES
Laparoscopic Nissen Fundoplication

The laparoscopic Nissen procedure is generally performed via the five (two 5 mm and three 10 mm) transabdominal ports positioned as described above, following the establishment of pneumoperitoneum, using a Veress needle introduced through an incision on a level with the No. 1 trocar site or the Hasson cannula when adhesions from previous surgery are expected. The surgeon stands between the patient's legs and handles the instruments through the two operative ports (Nos. 4 and 5), while the assistant on the right side holds the laparoscope and retracts the liver. The assistant on the left side retracts the stomach during esophageal dissection and raises the esophagus during access to the area behind the esophagus. This assistant also helps the surgeon during suturing procedures.

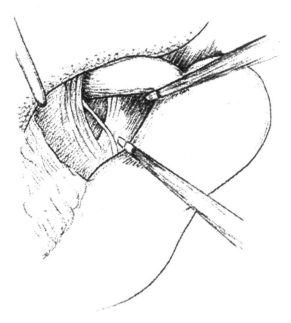

Fig. 5-4 Mobilization of the esophagus allows for the creation of a posterior window in the connective tissue just inferior to the left diaphragmatic crus. The posterior vagus nerve must be identified and separated from the posterior aspect of the esophagus.

The first step in the operation consists of vertically dividing the gastrohepatic ligament over a short distance along the upper lesser curvature of the stomach using the electrocautery hook and taking care to preserve the hepatic branches of the vagus nerve and to avoid bleeding from any aberrant left hepatic artery. Retraction of the stomach to the left side exposes the right diaphragmatic crus, which is dissected by gently incising the overlying peritoneum with the electrocautery hook or scissors. The right crus is dissected from the esophagus to give access to the posterior esophagus and to identify the crossing of the diaphragmatic crura. A similar dissection of the left crus is made after retraction of the stomach to the right side. The esophagus is elevated with a plastic tube to create a posterior window in the connective tissue just inferior to the left diaphragmatic crus (Fig. 5-4). Access to the cavity above the gastric fundus, which in the case of hiatal hernia is located in the mediastinum, is gained by gentle dissection that must not be extended too far upward to avoid damage to the left pleura, which would cause pneumothorax, mediastinal air tracking, and a subcutaneous neck emphysema. During this stage of the operation, dissection must not be performed too close to the posterior wall of the stomach and esophagus to avoid perforation. When the window behind the esophagus is created, the next step is to identify and dissect the right vagus nerve from the posterior wall of the esophagus because the gastric wrap must be positioned between the anterior aspect of the nerve and the posterior wall of the esophagus. A 50 to 60 F dilator is inserted in the esophagus prior to hiatoplasty, which consists of

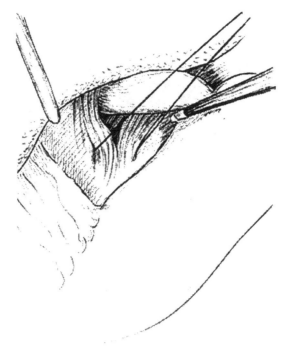

Fig. 5-5 Hiatoplasty involves one to three stitches passed from the left to the right diaphragmatic crus to allow crural closure. This step must be completed when a 50 to 60 F bougie is introduced into the esophagus to avoid esophageal dysphagia.

crural closure behind the esophagus and in front of the posterior vagus nerve, by means of one to three 2-0 monofilament sutures passed from the left to the right side through the muscle fibers of the diaphragmatic crura and tied using the extracorporeal knot-tying technique. The stitches must be passed and tied gently to avoid esophageal stricture and to ensure a crural closure sufficient to prevent the gastric fundoplication from slipping into the chest when the intraesophageal bougie is removed (Fig. 5-5).

The next step in the procedure involves mobilization of the upper 10 cm of the greater curvature of the stomach by clipping and dividing short gastric vessels and peritoneal attachments to the spleen and diaphragm (Fig. 5-6). This is not always necessary because the proximal part of the fundus often has long vascular and peritoneal attachments that do not interfere with fundoplication fashioning. In such cases, attention must be paid to avoid interposing the gastric fat pad between the esophagus and the gastric fundus because this would encourage slipping of the gastric wrap on the esophagus, especially when the Nissen-Rossetti technique is used. Following the reinsertion of the intraesophageal dilator, the mobilized gastric fundus is grasped with a clamp and passed through the window behind the esophagus from left to right to create a wrap around the intra-abdominal esophagus (Fig. 5-7). According to the classic Nissen technique, the gastric wrap must be total, that is, 360 degrees and 2 to 4 cm long. The limbs of the fundoplication should be fixed

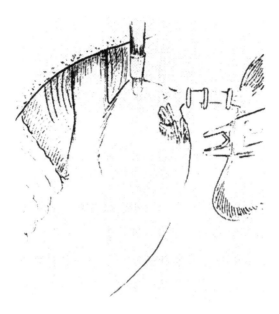

Fig. 5-6   The short gastric vessels are frequently clipped and divided to mobilize the gastric fundus necessary for fundoplication.

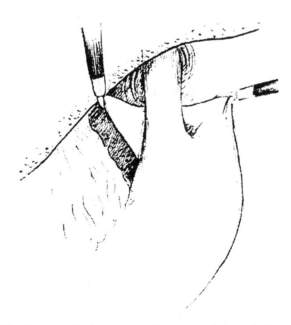

Fig. 5-7   The mobilized gastric fundus is grasped and passed through the window created behind the esophagus.

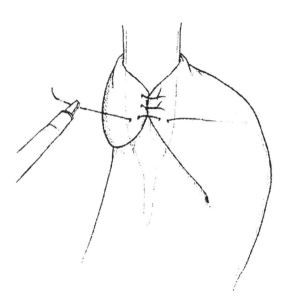

Fig. 5-8   The Nissen-Rossetti technique consists of creating a short loose posterior fundoplication that is not fixed to the anterior wall of the esophagus.

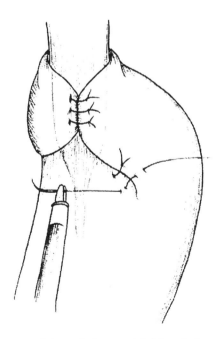

Fig. 5-9   One to two stitches passed through the wrap's left hemivalve and the anterior surface of the gastric body prevent gastric "telescoping" phenomenon.

with two or three sutures that pass through the anterior muscular wall of the esophagus. Knots can be tied either with the extracorporeal technique, using 2-0 long monofilament sutures, or with the intracorporeal technique, which uses 2-0 short silk sutures. Some authors use a single U-shaped stitch of 2-0 monofilament suture with two Teflon pledgets on the outer surface of each limb of the wrap to fix the fundoplication, plus two simple 2-0 monofilament sutures placed above and below the U stitch.[12] We prefer to fashion the fundoplication according to the Rossetti modification, which consists of a loose, floppy, 2 cm long total posterior gastric wrap that is not fixed to the anterior esophageal wall (Fig. 5-8). Gastric wrap "telescoping" is prevented by fixing the lower part of the wrap's left hemivalve to the anterior surface of the gastric body with one or two additional stitches (Fig. 5-9). Fundoplication tightness is controlled by replacing the dilator in the stomach. Finally, intraperitoneal liquids are aspirated and the pneumoperitoneum is released. Removal of the transabdominal ports is followed by closure of the small cutaneous incisions. Major defects in the muscle layers of the abdominal wall must be closed with absorbable transfascial sutures to avoid postoperative hernia formation.

Laparoscopic Toupet Fundoplication

Chronic gastroesophageal reflux may cause defective peristalsis in the esophageal distal body. Some patients with endoscopic grade II esophagitis show esophageal contractions with amplitudes below 30 mm Hg, while patients with more severe reflux esophagitis, Barrett's esophagus, or peptic stricture may present with no motility along the entire esophageal body.[37] Because Nissen fundoplication may also aggravate preexisting poor esophageal body function and dysphagia,[38] a posterior 270-degree gastric fundoplication, which can also be completed through a laparoscopic access, has been recommended to correct pathologic gastroesophageal reflux in patients with defective peristalsis.

The operative procedure is similar to the Nissen fundoplication, except that the posterior gastric wrap does not require fundus mobilization from the spleen. The fundoplication should be 3 to 4 cm long and fixed to the right and left margins of the anterior wall of the esophagus with two or three 2-0 monofilament sutures on each side, tied using the extracorporeal knot-tying technique (Fig. 5-10). This procedure emphasizes the angle of His and increases LES resting tone, albeit to a lesser degree than the Nissen technique.

Laparoscopic Dor Fundoplication

Dor fundoplication consists of an anterior gastric hemifundoplication that is usually performed to prevent iatrogenic gastroesophageal reflux in patients with primary esophageal achalasia after extramucosal Heller's myotomy.[39] Since dissection is limited during myotomy to the anterior wall of the esophagus, this antireflux procedure seems to be the most suitable, partly because it does not require wide dissection and because it protects the esophageal mucosa exposed by the myotomy. The procedure can be performed laparoscopically by suturing the anterior wall of

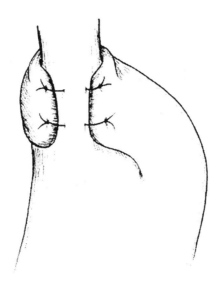

Fig. 5-10 Toupet fundoplication is a posterior 270-degree wrap. The gastric fundus is fixed to the lateral margins of the esophagus.

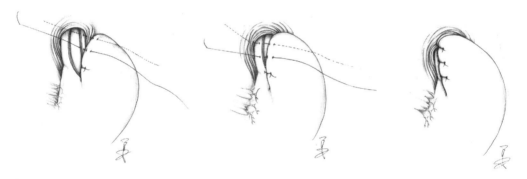

Fig. 5-11 The Dor operation is an anterior 180-degree fundoplication performed after myotomy for esophageal achalasia. The wrap is fixed to the lateral edges of the myotomy on both sides.

the gastric fundus, which is not mobilized from the spleen, to the edges of the myotomy with three nonabsorbable sutures on each side. The upper stitch includes the diaphragmatic crus and prevents the fundoplication from slipping into the chest (Fig. 5-11). The trocars are positioned in more or less the same way as for the other classic antireflux procedures, except that the trocar for the optic is located higher, on the midpoint of the xiphoid-umbilical line, so that the myotomy can be extended proximally into the mediastinum.

Laparoscopic Ligamentum Teres Cardiopexy

This original technique, described by Narbona-Arnau[40] and adapted for laparoscopy by Nathanson, Shimi, and Cuschieri[15] with some modifications regarding

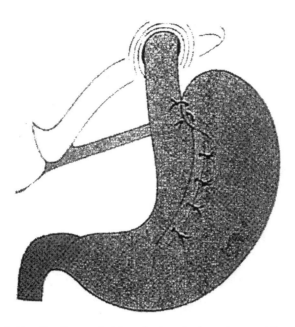

Fig. 5-12   Cardiopexy fashioned using the hepatic round ligament.

blood supply preservation of the ligament, has proved effective in achieving LES competence by lengthening its intra-abdominal segment, restoring the angle of His, and increasing the pressure in the high pressure zone. The procedure requires five trocars, two 11.5 mm and three 5.5 mm. The two 11.5 mm trocars are inserted just above the umbilicus, one on the right and one on the left, along the linea semi-lunaris. They are used for the insertion of the laparoscope and clip applicator. Three 5.5 mm trocar ports are used for the operating instruments. One is placed just below and to the right of the xiphoid process, one to the right of the midline halfway between the subxiphoid and the right 11.5 mm trocar, and one close to the lower end of the left costal margin.

The technique makes use of the round hepatic ligament to construct an intra-abdominal segment at the esophagogastric junction. This acts as a flutter valve when the anterior and posterior walls are apposed by intra-abdominal pressure rises. The first step is mobilization of the round hepatic ligament with preservation of its blood supply from the liver and peritoneal attachments, followed by mobi-lization of the intra-abdominal esophagus and fashioning of the cardiopexy using the round ligament (Fig. 5-12).

Laparoscopic Placement of the Angelchick Prosthesis

Trocar positioning and the mobilization of the intra-abdominal esophagus are the same as for the laparoscopic Nissen procedure. The silicon prosthesis is intro-duced through the No. 1 access after removal of the Hasson cannula. If the hiatal opening is large enough, a hiatoplasty is performed to prevent prosthesis herniation into the mediastinum. The prosthesis is passed through the window created behind

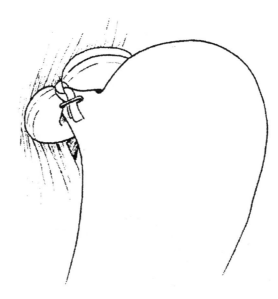

Fig. 5-13   The Angelchick prosthesis is placed laparoscopically as during open surgery.

the esophagus by posterior dissection. The vagus nerve can be left on the inside or outside of the prosthesis, which is then placed in the required position at the esophagogastric junction. A dilator bougie is inserted in the esophagus before intracorporeal tying of the Dacron straps with four knots. One or two metal clips are used to prevent the ends of the straps from coming undone. Some surgeons also secure the strap knot to the fatty tissue on the anterior surface of the stomach using an EndoLoop tie of absorbable material to prevent any dislocation of the prosthesis[16] (Fig. 5-13).

POSTOPERATIVE MANAGEMENT

Antireflux laparoscopic surgery offers a shorter postoperative course than conventional open laparotomy. In our experience, after an initial learning phase, during which the laparoscopic surgeon becomes familiar with the technique, postoperative management becomes standardized and free of complications. Postoperative antibiotics are not necessary. A preoperative short-term antibiotic prophylaxis is generally provided at the induction of anesthesia. No drains are placed unless there are intraoperative complications. A nasogastric tube is positioned and removed on the first or second postoperative day after a radiographic contrast study. Some authors do not use a nasogastric tube.[4,19] Patients are allowed to eat and are discharged on the third or fourth day with instructions to eat only soft foods. A mild transient dysphagia is usually present during the first month. Patients are seen 1 and 12 months after surgery for a clinical evaluation, and at 6 and 24 months for a full evaluation, including endoscopy, esophageal manometry, and 24-hour pH monitoring.

CASE SERIES AND RESULTS

Between June 1992 and December 1994, 24 patients with GERD diagnosed by esophageal 24-hour pH monitoring were selected for laparoscopic antireflux surgery. In three patients (12.5%), conversion to laparotomy was necessary to deal adequately with two paraesophageal hernias and one hiatal hernia. Nineteen Nissen-Rossetti and two Toupet procedures were performed. The average duration of the operation was 182 minutes (range, 118 to 243 minutes). Five patients had no endoscopic esophagitis, two had grade I esophagitis, seven had grade II, four had grade III, and three had Barrett's esophagus. No patient had a peptic stricture. Hiatal hernia was present in 17 patients, one of whom had an enormous mixed (hiatal plus paraesophageal) gastric herniation. No intraoperative major complications occurred during esophageal dissection, gastric mobilization, and wrap fashioning. A Silastic drain was positioned in the splenic region in five cases, at the cardia in four, and in the subhepatic region in two cases. Morbidity included two cases of slipped Nissen, one of which required an open reoperation on the third postoperative day, one case of dynamic ileus (treated conservatively), one case of pneumonia (requiring 13 days of hospitalization), one case of paroxysmal atrial fibrillation, which was converted pharmacologically with amiodarone (Cordarone) infusion, and two cases of transient subcutaneous emphysema of the chest and cervical region (Fig. 5-14). Antibiotics were used only for the patient who developed pneumonia. The use of analgesic drugs was limited and in the majority of cases was unnecessary. A nasogastric tube was routinely positioned in the first 19 patients and was avoided in the

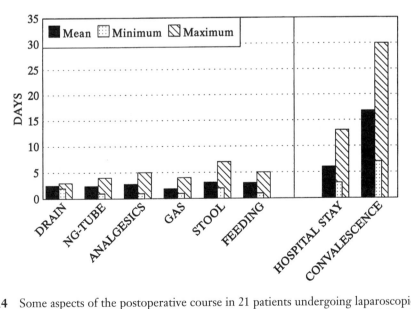

Fig. 5-14 Some aspects of the postoperative course in 21 patients undergoing laparoscopic Nissen-Rossetti fundoplication. In two patients (9.5%), no nasogastric tube was positioned. In 10 patients (48%), abdominal drainage was unnecessary. Five patients (24%) required no pain-relief medication in the postoperative period. Hospitalization was brief and a complete recovery to normal activity was achieved in 2 weeks.

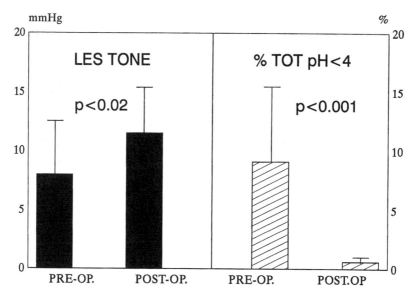

Fig. 5-15 A significant increase in LES resting pressure was obtained with the laparoscopic Nissen-Rossetti repair in the 16 patients who had postoperative manometry *(left)*. A significant decrease in the total percentage time of esophageal acid exposure was demonstrated with 24-hour esophageal pH monitoring *(right)*.

last two patients. The return to bowel transit and natural feeding was exceptionally good. The average hospital stay was 6 days (range, 3 to 13 days) with a mean convalescence of 17 days (range, 7 to 30 days) calculated on the basis of the time required to return to work or normal activity. A clinical follow-up of the 21 patients at a mean of 9.5 months (range, 1 to 25 months) was made. Two patients had severe dysphagia and one was reoperated on after 3 months by laparotomy because of an excessively tight hiatus. The other was successfully treated by means of two pneumatic dilations. No recurrent reflux symptoms were recorded (see Table 5-1). Repeated manometry and pH-monitoring, after a mean follow-up period of 7 months (range, 1 to 25 months), was performed on 16 patients. All patients had a significant increase in LES resting tone after laparoscopic surgery and there was no abnormal esophageal acid exposure (Fig. 5-15). Improved esophageal body motility and complete regression of esophagitis after a laparoscopic Toupet fundoplication was seen in one of the two patients who had preoperative esophageal peristaltic dysfunction. Endoscopy performed prior to postoperative functional studies in the 16 patients who completed the follow-up showed no signs of recurrent hiatal hernia or macroscopic esophagitis. The follow-up in one patient with Barrett's esophagus showed no regression.

DISCUSSION

Despite the recent introduction of new acid suppressants such as omeprazole, surgery still competes well with medical therapy for the treatment of GERD.[41] The

Table 5-2   Number of operations per year

Author	Laparotomy Era	Laparoscopic Era
Collard et al.[12,44]	23	26
DeMeester et al.[43]	24	23
DelGenio et al.[27]	12	15
Siewert et al.[45]	14	18
Ancona and Peracchia et al.[33,34,46,47]	11	12
Jamieson et al.[24,48]	10	62
Hinder et al.[14,49]	15	76
Boulez et al.[32]	?	53
Cadiere et al.[23]	?	59
Dallemagne et al.[6,19]	?	143

indications for surgery, manometrically detected LES deficiency and abnormal gastroesophageal reflux on 24-hour pH-monitoring, must be clearly defined. There are numerous antireflux techniques, but the Nissen procedure is probably superior for long-term reflux control.[10,42,43] Results after the laparoscopic approach were very similar to those of the open procedure and the technique used was the same as for the conventional open Nissen operation. Reports of published series of the laparoscopic treatment of GERD confirm that total posterior fundoplication (Nissen) is certainly the preferred procedure, albeit with technical variations from one surgeon to another. The rate of conversion to open surgery varies from 0% to 25% and this variability probably depends not only on the experience of the surgeon, but also on different attitudes to the possible need for conversion. Some surgeons report on the use of the laparoscopic approach to treat difficult cases with giant hiatal or paraesophageal hernias and convert to open surgery only in the event of uncontrollable intraoperative complications. Others convert to laparotomy more frequently, especially when anatomic difficulties prevent the completion of the procedure to perfection. Table 5-2 provides data from the literature and shows the difference in the number of antireflux operations performed yearly before and after the introduction of laparoscopy by various authors. Some authors continue to perform a similar number of operations each year, whereas others show a significant increase in the total number of antireflux repairs performed since the introduction of the laparoscopic technique. This increase could be related to a referral pattern to particular centers for less invasive treatment, or to a broadening of the indications for laparoscopic treatment.

Despite a significant decrease in the operative time with increasing experience,[14,19,24] the average duration of laparoscopic procedures is longer than the corresponding laparotomy techniques. The longer duration of the procedure does not seem to influence the morbidity and postoperative course, in which pain and discomfort are minimal and hospital stay and convalescence are shorter. The literature describes only a few cases of wound contamination after laparoscopic surgery, thus justifying the abandonment of the systemic use of postoperative antibiotic therapy. A preoperative short-term prophylaxis with 2 gm intravenous ceftriaxone is given

Table 5-3   Complications of laparoscopic antireflux surgery (1012 operations)

	No. of Patients	%
Subcutaneous emphysema (chest and neck)	30	2.9
Pneumothorax	13	1.3
Esophageal/gastric perforation	10	1.0
Pneumonia	9	0.9
Bleeding	8	0.8
Pulmonary embolism	7	0.7
Wrap slipping	4	0.4
Ileus	3	0.3
Cardiac arrhythmias	1	0.1
Intra-abdominal abscess	1	0.1
Other	8	0.8
Urinary infections	2	
Pleural effusion	1	
Wrap necrosis	1	
Aspiration	1	
Necrosing pancreatitis	1	
Bacteremia with jaundice	1	
ARDS	1	
	94	9.3

at the induction of general anesthesia. Judging from the larger case series,[14,19,24] the use of a nasogastric tube to prevent dilation linked to gastric paresis is also being discontinued. On the other hand, 12- to 24-hour nasogastric tube aspiration prevents gastric distention prior to the recovery of bowel movements and limits vomiting and excessive tension on the fundoplication. Drains are used only in the event of the risk of bleeding or iatrogenic tissue damage and only for very brief periods. Table 5-3 lists the most common complications of laparoscopic antireflux surgery in a series of 1012 operations, 981 of which (97%) were Nissen or Nissen-Rossetti procedures. The remaining 3% included a teres cardiopexy in nine cases, a Toupet procedure in 10 cases, a Dor procedure in 10 cases, and a Lortat-Jacob procedure in two cases.* Subcutaneous emphysema located in the chest and cervical regions in 2.9% of cases was due to carbon dioxide trapped in the mediastinum during dissection of the hiatal region when a window was made behind the esophagus. This emphysema is sometimes very severe and deforming, but is always transient and usually resolves spontaneously.[20,30] Pneumothorax occurred in 1.3% of patients and was linked to left pleural damage during dissection and hernia reduction. It may be minimal and recede spontaneously, but sometimes requires a chest aspiration tube. Moderate bleeding occurs during cardia dissection and is generally easy to control laparoscopically, but can sometimes be severe and may require conversion to laparotomy, especially when it is from an aberrant left hepatic artery during right crus

*References 12, 14, 19, 20, 23-25, 28, 30, 35, and 36.

dissection or from the gastrosplenic vasa brevia during gastric fundus mobilization. Perforation of viscera is another important cause of morbidity. There are no reports of organ damage caused by the insertion of trocars during laparoscopic antireflux procedures. Perforation generally occurs during the operative phases and involves the posterior aspect of the esophagus at the cardia during the creation of the posterior window, the stomach during fundus mobilization, the passage of the fundus behind the esophagus to create the wrap, or when the stomach is pulled down with traumatic forceps. The rare cases of pulmonary embolism reported after laparoscopic antireflux operations may not justify the routine use of low-dose heparin as prophylaxis for deep venous thrombosis, except for patients at risk. Other complications, which occur in a very small percentage of cases, are not strictly linked to the operative stages of the laparoscopic antireflux repair. In all published case series, hospitalization is brief. In the absence of complications, it never exceeds the fourth or fifth postoperative day. The average percentage of success of the various antireflux procedures in 21 series, including 1513 patients, amounts to 92.8% (range, 77% to 100%) (see Table 5-1). These results confirm the efficacy of the laparoscopic treatment of GERD. However, in most of the series, satisfactory results have been reported only on a subjective, clinical basis, without evaluation of the functional effects of the various antireflux plications. In our series, all patients underwent postoperative manometric and pH-monitoring studies that demonstrated an increase in LES pressure and a decrease in esophageal acid exposure, with complete regression of endoscopic esophagitis. In our opinion, postoperative results must always be considered in the light of functional studies, including postoperative manometry and 24-hour pH monitoring, especially in the long-term follow-up.

REFERENCES

1. Petelin JB. Laparoscopic approach to common duct pathology. Surg Laparosc Endosc 1:33-41, 1991.
2. Fitzgibbons RJ, Salerno G, Filipi CJ, Hunter WJ, Watson P. A laparoscopic intraperitoneal onlay mesh technique for the repair on an indirect inguinal hernia. Ann Surg 219:144-156, 1994.
3. Phillips EH, Franklin M, Carroll BJ, Fallas MJ, Ramos R, Rosenthal D. Laparoscopic colectomy. Ann Surg 216:703-707, 1992.
4. Soper NJ, Brunt LM, Fleshman J, Dunnegan DL, Cayman RV. Laparoscopic small bowel resection and anastomosis. Surg Laparosc Endosc 3:6-12, 1993.
5. Ancona E, Anselmino M, Zaninotto G, Costantini M, Rossi M, Bonavina L, Boccu C, Buin F, Peracchia A. Esophageal achalasia: Laparoscopic versus conventional open Heller-Dor operation. Am J Surg 1995 (in press).
6. Dallemagne B, Weerts JM, Jehaes C, Markiewicz S, Lombard R. Laparoscopic Nissen fundoplication: Preliminary report. Surg Laparosc Endosc 3:138-143, 1991.
7. Costantini M, Crookes PF, Bremner RM, Hoeft SF, Ehsan A, Peters JH, Bremner CG, DeMeester TR. Value of physiologic assessment of foregut symptoms in a surgical practice. Surgery 114:780-787, 1993.
8. Zaninotto G, DeMeester TR, Scwizer W, Johansson KE, Cheng SC. The lower esophageal sphincter in health and disease. Am J Surg 155:104-111, 1988.
9. DeMeester TR. Surgical management of gastroesophageal reflux. In Castell DO, Wu WC, Ott DJ, eds. Gastroesophageal Reflux Disease: Pathogenesis, Diagnosis and Therapy. New York: Futura Publishing Co., 1985, pp 243-280.

10. DeMeester TR, Johnson LF, Kent AH. Evaluation of current operations for the prevention of gastroesophageal reflux. Ann Surg 180:511-525, 1974.
11. Geagea T. Laparoscopic Nissen's fundal plication is feasible. Can J Surg 34:313, 1991.
12. Collard JM, de Gheldere CA, De Kock M, Otte JB, Kestens PJ. Laparoscopic anti-reflux surgery. What is the real progress? Ann Surg 220:146-154, 1994.
13. Hinder RA, Filipi CJ. The technique of laparoscopic Nissen fundoplication. Surg Laparosc Endosc 2:265-267, 1992.
14. Hinder RA, Filipi CJ, Wetscher G, Neary P, DeMeester TR, Perdikis G. Laparoscopic Nissen fundoplication is an effective treatment for gastroesophageal reflux disease. Ann Surg 220:472-483, 1994.
15. Nathanson LK, Shimi S, Cuschieri A. Laparoscopic ligamentum teres (round ligamentum) cardiopexy. Br J Surg 78:947-951, 1991.
16. Berguer R, Stiegmann GU, Yamamoto M. Minimal access surgery for gastroesophageal reflux: Laparoscopic placement of the Angelchick prosthesis in pigs. Surg Endosc 5:123-126, 1991.
17. Lind JF, Duthie HL, Schlegel JR, Code CF. Motility of the gastric fundus. Am J Physiol 201:197-202, 1961.
18. Bagnato VJ. Laparoscopic Nissen fundoplication. Surg Laparosc Endosc 2:188-190, 1992.
19. Weerts JM, Dallemagne B, Hamoir E, Demarche M, Markiiewicz S, Jehaes C, Lombard R, Demoulin JC, Etienne M, Ferron PE, Fontaine F, Gillard V, Deforge M. Laparoscopic Nissen fundoplication: Detailed analysis of 132 patients. Surg Laparosc Endosc 3:359-364, 1993.
20. Cuschieri A. Laparoscopic anti-reflux surgery and repair of hiatal hernia. World J Surg 17:40-45, 1993.
21. Mutter D, Evrard S, Vix M, Keller P, Mendoza-Burgos L, Marescaux J. Laparoscopic Nissen-Rossetti fundoplication: 10 cases. La Presse Medicale 22:771-773, 1993.
22. MacPhee WM. The laparoscopic placement of the Angelchick anti-reflux prosthesis. Min Invas Ther 2:5-9, 1993.
23. Cadiere GB, Houben JJ, Bruyns J, Himpens J, Panzer JM, Galin M. Laparoscopic Nissen fundoplication: Technique and preliminary results. Br J Surg 81:400-403, 1994.
24. Jamieson GG, Watson DI, Britten-Jones R, Mitchell PC, Anvari M. Laparoscopic Nissen fundoplication. Ann Surg 220:137-145, 1994.
25. Bittner HB, Meyers WC, Brazer SR, Pappas TN. Laparoscopic Nissen fundoplication: Operative results and short-term follow-up. Am J Surg 167:193-200, 1994.
26. Materia A, Genco A, Spaziani E, Caruso C, DeLeo A, Neri T, Rossini B, Basso N. Gastro-oesophageal reflux disease: Surgical treatment by laparoscopy. Chir Endosc 11:(a)11, 1994.
27. DelGenio A, Maffettone V, Landolfi V, Izzo G, Di Martino N, Fei L, Cosenza A, Martella A. Nissen fundoplication through laparoscopy for the cure of gastro-esophageal reflux (GER). Chir Endosc 11:(a)12, 1994.
28. Cady J. Traitement coeliochirurgical des hernies hiatales et des reflux gastrooesophagiens. A propos de 150 cas. Chir Endosc 11:(a)15, 1994.
29. Hallerback B, Glise H, Johansson B. Results of laparoscopic Rossetti fundoplication. Gut 35(S4): A166, 1994.
30. Hallerback B, Glise H, Johansson B, Radmark T. Laparoscopic Rossetti fundoplication. Surg Endosc 8:1417-1422, 1994.
31. Feussner H, Stein HJ. Laparoscopic antireflux surgery and cardiomyotomy. Dis Esoph 7:17-23, 1994.
32. Boulez J, Espalieu PH, Fontaumard E. Laparoscopic Nissen-Rossetti fundoplication: Experience with 117 cases. Surg Endosc 8:943-032A, 1994.
33. Fingerhut A, Pacquet JC, Magdeleinat P, Etienne JC, Hay JM, and the Laparoscopic Working Committee for the French Associations for Research in Surgery. Laparoscopic Nissen fundoplication: Evaluation of feasibility. Surg Endosc 8:943-034A, 1994.
34. Peracchia A, Fumagalli U, Rosati R, Bonavina L, Bona S. Minimally invasive surgery for diseases of the esophagus. Intern J Surg Sci 1:19-21, 1994.

35. Ancona E, Costantini M, Zaninotto G, Anselmino M, Boccu C. Reflusso gastro-esofageo: Terapia laparoscopica. In Falcetto G, ed. Giornate Chirurgiche Biellesi, 1994, pp 35-41.
36. Ancona E, Costantini M, Zaninotto G, Anselmino M, Rossi M. Laparoscopic surgery for gastroesophageal reflux: The situation in Italy. Surg Endosc 1995 (in press).
37. Bremner RM, DeMeester TR, Crookes PF, Costantini M, Hoeft SF, Peters JH, Hagen J. The effect of symptoms and nonspecific motility abnormalities on outcomes of surgical therapy for gastroesophageal reflux disease. J Thorac Cardiovasc Surg 107:1244-1250, 1994.
38. Thor KBA, Silander T. Long-term randomized prospective trial of the Nissen procedure versus a modified Toupet technique. Ann Surg 210:719-724, 1989.
39. Bonavina L, Nosadini L, Bardini R, Beassato M, Peracchia A. Primary treatment of esophageal achalasia. Long-term results of myotomy and Dor fundoplication. Arch Surg 127:222-226, 1992.
40. Narbona-Arnau B. Pexy with the round ligament: The sling approach. In Siewert JR, Holscher AH, eds. Diseases of the Esophagus. Berlin, Heidelberg, New York: Springer, 1988, pp 1172-1177.
41. Spechler SJ, and the Department of Veterans Affairs Gastroesophageal Reflux Disease Study Group #277. Comparison of medical and surgical therapy for complicated gastroesophageal reflux disease in veterans. N Engl J Med 326:786-792, 1992.
42. Leonardi HK, Lee ME, El-Kurd MF, Ellis FH. An experimental study of the effectiveness of various anti-reflux operations. Ann Thorac Surg 24:215-222, 1977.
43. DeMeester TR, Bonavina L, Albertucci M. Nissen fundoplication for gastroesophageal reflux disease. Evaluation of primary repair in 100 consecutive patients. Ann Surg 204:9-20, 1986.
44. Collard JM, DeKoninck XJ, Otte JB, Fiasse RH, Kestens PJ. Intrathoracic Nissen fundoplication: Long-term clinical and pH-monitoring evaluation. Ann Thorac Surg 51:34-38, 1991.
45. Siewert JR, Feussner H, Walker SJ. Fundoplication: How to do it? Peri-esophageal wrapping as a therapeutic principal of gastroesophageal reflux prevention. World J Surg 16:326-334, 1992.
46. Zaninotto G, Costantini M, Anselmino M, Boccu C, Bagolin F, Polo R, Ancona E. Excessive competence of the lower esophageal sphincter after Nissen fundoplication: Evaluation by three-dimensional computerized imaging. Eur J Surg 1995 (in press).
47. Peracchia A, Bonavina L, Merigliano S, Anselmino M, Bardini R. Malattia da reflusso gastro-esofageo: Criteri di terapia chirurgica. In Montori A, DeAnna L, eds. Fifth International Symposium of Digestive Surgery and Endoscopy. Rome, Bologna: Monduzzi Ed, 1989, pp 165-172.
48. Jamieson GG. The results of antireflux surgery and reoperative antireflux surgery. Gullet 3:41-45, 1993.
49. Hinder RA, Stein HJ, Bremner CG, DeMeester TR. Relationship of a satisfactory outcome to normalization of a delayed gastric emptying after Nissen fundoplication. Ann Surg 210:458-465, 1989.

6

Infectious Esophagitis: Etiology, Diagnosis, and Treatment

Fabrizio Parente, M.D. • *Gabriele Bianchi Porro, M.D.*

Infectious esophagitis has been recognized for decades, but has only recently received direct attention in the medical literature. The condition is uncommon in immunocompetent subjects and, until the advent of endoscopy, could not be diagnosed antemortem with certainty, but could be suspected on the basis of radiographic findings. Flexible esophagoscopy permits direct visualization and biopsy of the esophagus. With the advent of immunosuppressive therapy, opportunistic infections of the esophagus have become more frequent. Knowledge of these conditions has escalated since the emergence of the human immunodeficiency virus (HIV) infection and its related diseases. Today, esophageal infections constitute one of the major causes of morbidity in patients with acquired immunodeficiency syndrome (AIDS) and have stimulated continued interest in their diagnosis and treatment.

This chapter summarizes the etiology of infectious esophagitis in immunocompetent and immunodeficient hosts, discusses the diagnostic strategies currently available, and reviews the recent advancements in treatment and prophylaxis.

ESOPHAGEAL INFECTIONS IN THE CONTEXT OF AIDS

Infections of the esophagus are very common in patients with HIV infection. Both retrospective[1,2] and prospective[3-5] studies have documented that 21% to 35% of HIV-infected patients complain of esophageal symptoms (mainly dysphagia and odynophagia) that are for the most part sustained by infections. They are important not only because of their frequency, but also because if untreated they may severely compromise the nutritional status of these patients and may be responsible for life-threatening complications. In addition, the development of an opportunistic esophagitis may be a marker of a poor prognosis, reflecting a more severe underlying immunodeficiency.[3,6,7] Almost all of these conditions are now potentially treatable so the correct diagnosis has important clinical implications.

Etiology

The complete spectrum of opportunistic pathogens that may be responsible for esophageal infection in HIV-infected patients is reported in Table 6-1. It must be emphasized that only anecdotal reports exist for many of these infections (especially the bacterial and parasitic) and most of the infections are sustained by fungi or viruses.

Esophageal Candidiasis

Candida esophagitis is the most frequent infection of the esophagus in patients with AIDS. In three large prospective studies on the frequency of esophageal diseases in HIV-infected patients referred to gastroenterologists for dysphagia and

Table 6-1 Spectrum of organisms responsible for esophageal infections in HIV-infected patients

Fungal	Bacterial
Candida albicans	Gram-positive coccobacilli
Candida krusei	Actinomycosis
Candida glabrata	*Mycobacterium avium-intracellulare*
Candida parapsilosis	*Mycobacterium tuberculosis*
Candida guilliermondii	
Histoplasmosis	**Protozoal**
Exophiala jeanselmei	
	Cryptosporidium
	Pneumocystis carinii
Viral	
Cytomegalovirus (CMV)	
Herpes simplex virus (HSV)	
Epstein-Barr virus	
Human immunodeficiency virus (HIV)	

Table 6-2 Frequency of the major esophageal lesions in HIV-infected patients

Authors	Year	No. of *Candida* sp (%)	No. of CMV (%)	No. of HSV (%)	No. of Kaposi's Sarcoma (%)	No. of Noninfectious Ulcerations (%)	No Lesions (%)
Connolly et al.[3] (n = 48)	1989	38 (79)	4 (8)	4 (8)	7 (15)	3 (6)	4 (8)
Bonacini et al.[5] (n = 110)	1991	57 (52)	31 (28)	10 (9)	1 (1)	6 (18)	37 (34)
Parente et al.[8] (n = 49)	1991	24 (49)	5 (10)	8 (16)	1 (2)	8 (16)	5 (10)

CMV = cytomegalovirus; HSV = herpes simplex virus.

odynophagia,[3,5,8] *Candida* esophagitis accounted for 49% to 79% of the symptoms (Table 6-2). However, 20% to 25% of patients had multiple diagnoses, mainly co-infection with *Candida* species and viruses.

Although *C. albicans* is the most common fungal pathogen, other *Candida* species, including *C. glabrata*, *C. Krusei*, and *C. guilliermondii*, have been reported in oroesophageal diseases.[9] Other reported fungal organisms resulting in symptomatic esophagitis include *Histoplasma capsulatum*[10] and *Exophiala jeanselmei*.[11]

Viral Esophagitis

Viral infections represent the second most common cause of esophagitis in the HIV-positive population. Members of the herpes virus family may sustain esophageal infections, including cytomegalovirus (CMV), herpes simplex virus (HSV), and Epstein-Barr virus. CMV infection has been reported in 10% to 28% of HIV-infected patients complaining of esophageal symptoms[3,5,8] and is frequently associated with an extraesophageal localization (retinitis, colitis).[12] HSV esophagitis (mainly caused by HSV type 1), which is not exclusive to immunosuppressed patients, is less common and is diagnosed in approximately 10% of HIV-infected patients (Table 6-2). Epstein-Barr virus has also been reported as a cause of esophagitis in these patients. DNA in situ hybridization studies revealed Epstein-Barr virus infection in five patients with esophageal ulcers.[13] However, additional studies are needed to evaluate the clinical relevance of this infection.

Esophageal ulcerations have also been described in patients with seroconversion to HIV.[14,15] These patients present with a "flu-like" illness and associated dysphagia or odynophagia. Endoscopic evaluation may reveal esophageal ulcers in which no specific pathogen can be identified. Since retroviral particles were revealed by electron microscopic examination of esophageal mucosal specimens, HIV has been suggested as the primary cause of these ulcers.

Bacterial Esophagitis

Bacteria appear to be an unusual cause of esophageal disease in patients with AIDS, although they may be responsible for esophagitis in patients with hematologic malignancies and diabetes. Invasive gram-positive bacteria have been found in one patient with AIDS presenting with odynophagia and erosive changes of the distal esophagus.[16]

Despite the common occurrence of pulmonary and systemic infection, *Mycobacterium avium-intracellulare* has been reported infrequently as a cause of esophageal symptoms[17] and *M. tuberculosis* is also rarely responsible for esophageal infection in AIDS patients.[18]

Protozoal Esophagitis

Despite the high frequency of protozoal infections of the gastrointestinal tract in HIV-infected patients, protozoal esophagitis has been reported infrequently.

The causative pathogens identified include *Cryptosporidium*[19] and *Pneumocystis carinii*.[20]

Other Conditions

Idiopathic chronic esophageal ulcers are being recognized more frequently in patients with AIDS. By definition, an esophageal ulceration in the setting of an HIV infection may be considered idiopathic only when thorough histopathologic examination of biopsy specimens from the lesion has excluded other causes. Recently Kotler et al.[21] reported on 12 cases of chronic idiopathic ulcers in patients with AIDS. HIV was found in all ulcers through the use of a combination of RNA in situ hybridization, immunohistochemistry, and antigen capture enzyme-linked immunosorbent assay of tissue homogenates, suggesting that these ulcers are caused by a direct cytopathic effect of HIV infection.

Diagnosis
Clinical Findings

Esophageal infections are usually manifested by the presence of esophageal symptoms, specifically dysphagia or odynophagia. There is not a clear relationship between the type of esophageal symptom and the cause of infectious esophagitis,[3,5] although the abrupt onset of odynophagia in the absence of dysphagia, as well as a spontaneous recurrent substernal pain, is more suggestive of ulcerative esophagitis (viral; idiopathic).[22] In contrast, patients with *Candida* esophagitis, when symptomatic, tend to present with dysphagia alone or dysphagia and odynophagia. In rare cases, the initial manifestation of an infectious esophagitis may be a complication such as acute upper gastrointestinal bleeding[23] or spontaneous esophageal perforation.[24]

Evaluation of the oropharynx may provide clues to the underlying esophageal infection, and oropharyngeal candidiasis may be a marker for concomitant esophageal disease, especially when associated with esophageal symptoms. Large reported series have shown that the positive predictive value of oral thrush and dysphagia or odynophagia for candidal esophagitis varies from 71% to 100%.[3,5,25] However, in our experience, oropharyngeal candidiasis is often absent in patients who have received topical antifungals and candidal esophagitis (especially grades I and II) may be completely asymptomatic. Therefore, although the presence of oral thrush in an HIV-infected patient with esophageal symptoms is highly suggestive of esophageal candidiasis, this association cannot always be considered diagnostic. In addition, 20% to 25% of HIV-infected patients with esophageal symptoms have multiple diagnoses, mainly coinfection with *Candida* sp and other treatable viruses.[3,5,8]

Oral and perioral herpetic infection may suggest underlying HSV esophagitis in HIV-infected patients who complain of esophageal symptoms, but the frequency of this association is variable.

Diagnostic Procedures
Serology

Although serologic tests for *Candida*, CMV, and HSV infection are currently available, they play no role in the diagnosis of esophageal infections. The rate of seropositivity for CMV and HSV is very high, especially in homosexual men in whom it may approach 100%. Therefore, a positive serologic test is too nonspecific to give a diagnostic clue.

Radiography

Double-contrast barium esophagography has a high sensitivity (over 80%) in detecting esophageal lesions and the radiographic appearance of the most common opportunistic causes of esophageal diseases have been well described.[26] However, the radiographic abnormalities are often nonspecific and endoscopy with biopsies and/or brushing is necessary to make a definite diagnosis. This has been well documented in a recent study by Connolly et al.,[27] who compared double-contrast esophagography prospectively with endoscopy in 43 HIV-infected patients who had esophageal symptoms. The barium esophagogram was interpreted as abnormal in only 50% of patients who had an esophageal-established diagnosis (endoscopy and biopsies) and in only 25% of the cases was the radiologic diagnosis correct.

Endoscopy With Biopsies and Cultures

There is no doubt that esophagoscopy, which provides direct visualization of the esophageal mucosa, as well as the ability to obtain specimens for histology, cytology, and cultures, constitutes the gold standard in the diagnosis of esophageal infections. Initially, there was some hesitation regarding the use of standard endoscopes in HIV-infected patients because of the possibility of HIV transmission through contaminated endoscopes and the potential exposure of endoscopic personnel. The standardization of disinfection procedures, along with the use of endoscope-washing machines and protective measures for endoscopy personnel, has eliminated these concerns.[28]

Esophageal candidiasis at endoscopy is suggested by the presence of white plaques with hyperemia, occasionally accompanied by ulcerations. According to Kodsi et al.,[29] the endoscopic appearance may be characterized as follows: grade I, few raised plaques up to 2 mm in size with hyperemia, but no ulceration; grade II, multiple raised plaques greater than 2 mm with hyperemia, but no ulcerations; grade III, confluent, elevated plaques, involving almost all of the mucosa, with hyperemia and ulcerations; and grade IV, similar to grade III, but with no spared mucosa and with a narrowed lumen. Although the endoscopic appearance is characteristic, definite confirmation can be made by finding *Candida* sp pseudohypha on biopsy and/or brushings. Direct examination of smears obtained by brushing has been reported to be more sensitive than histology in the diagnosis of candidiasis and this is probably due to the possibility of mycelium losses during the processing of fixed and embedded biopsy specimens.[25]

Endoscopic findings in CMV esophagitis are variable. In most of the cases solitary or multiple large ulcerations, mainly in the middle upper esophagus, are visible, but sometimes exudative esophagitis and polypoid masses can be found.[5,8] The need to detect characteristic large intranuclear inclusions on biopsy specimens to make the diagnosis is debatable. According to some authors, this manifestation is an essential hallmark of this type of esophagitis, and biopsies should be taken from the ulcer bed instead of from the edges because CMV infects stroma cells rather than epithelial cells.[30] In contrast, other authors do not consider this to be a condition "sine qua non" but consider a positive viral culture associated with endoscopic lesions sufficient to make a diagnosis of CMV esophagitis.[5] However, viral cultures are difficult to perform, require several days to read positive, and positivity may simply result from viremia, with blood contamination from the biopsy specimen.

HSV esophagitis typically results in multiple shallow ulcerations, although the lesions may be confluent, causing an extensive erosive esophagitis that may be difficult to differentiate from other types of esophagitis (i.e., CMV or *Candida*). Vesicles are rarely seen. The definite diagnosis depends on mucosal biopsy and culture or cytologic examination of esophageal brushings from these lesions.[31]

Chronic idiopathic esophageal ulcers are usually giant and deep ulcers (>2 cm), located in the middle upper esophagus, that may appear endoscopically similar to CMV ulcerations. By definition, their diagnosis requires that a thorough histopathologic examination of biopsy specimens taken from the lesion is negative for infectious or neoplastic causes.[21]

Blind Esophageal Brushing

A minimally invasive technique has recently been proposed for the diagnosis of *Candida* esophagitis. A sterile brush is inserted through, and extended along, a nasogastric tube positioned in the esophagus, which makes it possible to obtain esophageal brushings that can be evaluated both cytologically and with appropriate fungal staining. When compared to parendoscopic brushing, this technique revealed comparable sensitivity for the diagnosis of *Candida* esophagitis.[32] It is, however, not useful in the diagnosis of other concomitant esophageal disorders or viral infections.

Treatment
Candida Esophagitis

Topical antifungals (i.e., nystatin) have some efficacy against oropharyngeal candidiasis but are less likely to cure esophageal infection. Recently, a small open trial on 25 men with AIDS showed that clotrimazole vaginal tablets taken orally are effective against *Candida* esophagitis.[33] Oral miconazole, supplied in a gel formulation, also appeared to be efficacious in a small study.[34] Further confirmation is needed before these treatments can be recommended for routine use. At present,

Table 6-3 Recommended regimens for treatment of common esophageal infections

Infection	Treatment
Candidiasis	Ketoconazole (200 to 400 mg/day) Fluconazole (100 to 150 mg/day) × 21 days Itraconazole (100 mg/day) Amphotericin B (0.3 mg/kg/day) maximum total dose 500 mg
Herpes simplex virus	Acyclovir (IV: 15 mg/kg/day; PO: 200 to 400 mg 5×day) × 14 to 21 days
Cytomegalovirus	Ganciclovir (induction: 5 mg/kg/b.i.d. × 14 to 21 days; maintenance: 6 mg/kg/day, 5 to 7 days/week) Foscarnet (60 mg/kg/day q8h or 90 mg/kg/b.i.d. × 14 to 21 days)

the most commonly used agents for *Candida* esophagitis in patients with AIDS are ketoconazole and fluconazole (Table 6-3). Ketoconazole in a daily dosage of 200 to 400 mg has been shown to be very effective in the short-term therapy of esophageal candidiasis in many uncontrolled series, with success rates of 50% to 70% after 3 to 4 weeks of therapy.[22] The efficacy of fluconazole (in daily dosage of 100 to 150 mg) against ketoconazole has been confirmed recently in a large, double-blind, multicenter comparative trial.[35] After 8 weeks of therapy, 100 mg/day of fluconazole resulted in a significantly higher rate of both symptomatic improvement (85% vs. 65%), endoscopic cure of esophageal candidiasis (91% vs. 52%), and a faster resolution of esophageal symptoms than 200 mg/day of ketoconazole. Both agents proved to be safe and well tolerated. A new azole congener, itraconazole, has recently become available. Smith et al.[36] compared 200 mg itraconazole, given once daily, with 200 mg ketoconazole, given twice daily, in the short-term therapy of both oropharyngeal and esophageal candidiasis. After 4 weeks of therapy the clinical response rate was 93% for both groups, but itraconazole was better tolerated. Only one patient discontinued itraconazole for toxicity compared to five patients taking ketoconazole. Treatment failures of short-term oral antifungals can occur, although the frequency and mechanisms are poorly understood. In a recent report,[8] almost all patients with esophageal candidiasis refractory to standard doses of oral ketoconazole or fluconazole subsequently improved with stronger antifungal therapy (increasing daily doses of fluconazole, intravenous fluconazole, or amphotericin B). Due to its high toxicity, it is usual to reserve amphotericin B for those patients who do not respond to high-dose intravenous fluconazole.

Virtually all patients with AIDS experience a relapse of esophageal candidiasis within 12 months from the first episode.[37] Given the efficacy of the prophylactic regimen with ketoconazole and fluconazole in immunosuppressed patients undergoing chemotherapy, antifungal prophylaxis may also be considered for HIV-infected patients after the resolution of the first episode of candidiasis. A recent study has confirmed that low doses of ketoconazole (200 mg/day) and fluconazole (50 mg/day) are effective in reducing the recurrence rates of esophageal candidiasis in patients with AIDS. However, relapses were frequently not responsive to full doses of the same antifungals, probably because of the development of resistant *Candida* organisms.[37] Therefore, the potential benefit of a prophylactic antifungal regimen must be evaluated against the risk of inducing resistance and the high cost of treatment. At present, in our experience, a maintenance antifungal treatment can be suggested only for patients with proved frequent symptomatic relapses.

Cytomegalovirus Esophagitis

Two parenteral agents have proved to be effective in the treatment of CMV infection, ganciclovir and foscarnet. Uncontrolled studies have shown that the response rate to ganciclovir for all forms of CMV gastrointestinal infections is approximately 79%.[38] In the largest uncontrolled series reported on foscarnet and ganciclovir,[39] the response rate was similar (77%). Foscarnet also appeared to be efficacious in patients whose gastrointestinal disease failed to respond to ganciclovir.[40] The preliminary results of a multicenter Italian study comparing ganciclovir with foscarnet in the treatment of CMV esophagitis were recently reported.[41] After 21 days of therapy, endoscopic improvement was observed in 73% of patients treated with foscarnet and 78% of patients treated with ganciclovir. Symptomatic relief was also similar with both drugs (91% and 89%, respectively) and no significant difference in the rate of side effects was noted. Therefore, given the different toxicity of the two compounds, the choice of anti-CMV drug should be individualized. Patients with impaired renal function or those receiving nephrotoxic drugs are better treated with ganciclovir. By contrast, for patients with neutropenia, foscarnet should be given as the drug of choice.

HSV Esophagitis

This infection is not exclusive to immunosuppressed patients, but can occur in otherwise healthy individuals. In these patients the disease is usually self-limiting and complete symptom resolution occurs within 10 to 12 days from the onset. In HIV-infected patients, it is more severe and requires specific antiviral therapy. The standard course of therapy with acyclovir in these patients appears to be effective,[3,8] but the need for prophylactic therapy after a successful acute course is debatable. Currently, these patients are treated with intravenous acyclovir for 3 weeks or until symptom resolution and then maintained with clinical observation only.

Idiopathic Esophageal Ulcers

These ulcers appear to be responsive, at least in the short-term period, to high-dose systemic steroid therapy. In a recent series of 12 patients with AIDS and chronic idiopathic esophageal ulcers, oral or intravenous steroids produced pain relief and weight gain in 10 patients.[21] On the basis of this and his own experience, Wilcox[22] has proposed the use of short-term oral steroids (a 1-month course of prednisone, 40 mg/day, tapering to 10 mg/wk) in patients with well-established idiopathic ulcers. Such short-term treatment therapy with steroids has not increased the incidence of other systemic or local infections.

INFECTIONS IN IMMUNOCOMPETENT HOSTS

Infectious esophagitis in immunocompetent subjects is unusual. The most commonly reported infections in the absence of any predisposing factor are probably HSV and *Candida* esophagitis. Shortsleeve and Levine[42] reported recently on a series of five otherwise healthy male patients with HSV esophagitis and no underlying immunologic problems. In all patients the predominant clinical manifestation was acute dysphagia that developed after a "flu-like" prodromal syndrome. All patients had an acute self-limiting illness, with complete symptom resolution within 10 to 12 days from the onset.[42]

Another infection that may occur in apparently healthy individuals is esophageal candidiasis. In most cases, however, some local or systemic factors predisposing to the infection may be recognized, including antibiotic treatment, the use of inhaled corticosteroids, and the use of potent antisecretory drugs (H_2 blockers, proton pump inhibitors). Alcoholism, malnutrition, and advanced age have also been associated with an increased risk of developing *Candida* esophagitis,[43] although these conditions probably predispose to infection through immunologic changes. Esophageal motility disorders may also predispose to candidiasis. Approximately one third of patients with scleroderma who undergo endoscopy have esophageal candidiasis.[44] Other disorders associated with candidiasis are diabetes mellitus, achalasia, and all the causes of esophageal obstruction.[45] The management of candidiasis in these individuals does not significantly differ from that of patients with HIV infection, although the response rate to antifungals tends to be higher and the recurrence rate is lower.

Another rare infection of the esophageal mucosa in the nonimmunocompromised host is *M. tuberculosis*. It is generally secondary to oral ingestion of the bacteria or to the involvement from adjacent infected mediastinal lymph nodes.

Recently, Mokoena et al.[46] reported on 11 cases of esophageal tuberculosis seen over a period of 18 years. The most common presenting symptom was dysphagia (nine cases), although two patients presented with massive hematemesis. The most important differential diagnosis was esophageal carcinoma because endoscopy revealed an ulcerating mass or polypoid tumor in 30% of the cases. Diagnosis was made by endoscopic esophageal biopsy in 50% of the cases and either biopsy of associated mediastinal or cervical lymph node masses or the presence of acid-fast bacilli in the sputum. Of the 10 patients who were managed by conventional antituberculosis drug treatment, nine had an uneventful recovery, but one died from hemorrhage from an aorta-esophageal fistula.

INFECTIONS IN OTHER IMMUNOSUPPRESSED PATIENTS

Patients with malignancy and those receiving organ transplantation are usually immunosuppressed and are at risk for opportunistic esophageal infections, although the latter are less frequent than infections in other organs (i.e., pneumonitis). Esophageal infections in these populations are mainly caused by *Candida* sp, CMV, and HSV. Prospective studies in diabetics undergoing renal transplantation reported a 2.2% incidence of *Candida* esophagitis,[47] but no significant correlation was established between the dosage of immunosuppressive agents and the frequency of esophageal infection. Another prospective study on liver and renal transplant recipients undergoing endoscopy for dysphagia or odynophagia found viral esophagitis in 11% of patients, with an equivalent percentage of CMV and HSV.[48] The treatment of esophageal infection in this setting follows the protocol adopted for HIV-infected patients. However, long-term suppressive therapy with antiviral agents in transplantation recipients is rarely necessary because the leukocyte count returns to normal after chemotherapy or reduction of immunosuppressive agents. Moreover, all of the potential measures to prevent CMV infection in patients undergoing transplantation should be adopted. These measures include testing for CMV of both the donor and the recipient and antiviral prophylaxis (ganciclovir, 5 mg/kg twice daily for 5 days, then once daily for 100 days) for seropositive recipients or those who receive organs from seropositive donors.[49]

RECOMMENDATIONS FOR DIAGNOSIS AND TREATMENT IN THE HIV SETTING

In HIV-infected patients with esophageal symptoms, the initial evaluation should include (1) an adequate characterization of symptoms (dysphagia, odynophagia, retrosternal pain, symptoms suggestive of reflux), as well as the evaluation of their severity; (2) a determination of the severity of immunodeficiency state (if the CD4 count is less than 100, an opportunistic esophageal infection is highly probable); (3) the presence of oral thrush, which may be suggestive of *Candida* esophagitis; and (4) the use of potentially esophagotoxic drugs (i.e., zidovudine, tetracycline).

Given these factors and taking into account the great preponderance of *Candida* esophagitis over the other forms of infection, the following guidelines are suggested. For patients presenting with mild to moderate esophagitis, and especially if they have a concomitant oral thrush, an empiric short-course treatment with antifungal medication (ketoconazole, fluconazole) is indicated. If rapid symptomatic relief occurs, treatment should be continued for at least 14 to 21 days to eradicate the infection. If symptoms persist after 8 to 10 days of therapy, an upper gastrointestinal endoscopy should be done to provide a definite diagnosis. In patients presenting with severe dysphagia or odynophagia, and oral intake is limited, esophagoscopy should be performed at an early stage to make a diagnosis and begin appropriate therapy.

REFERENCES

1. Gelb A, Miller S. AIDS and gastroenterology. Am J Gastroenterol 81:619-622, 1986.
2. May GR, Gill MJ, Church DL, et al. Gastrointestinal symptoms in ambulatory HIV-infected patients. Dig Dis Sci 38:1388-1394, 1993.
3. Connolly GM, Hawkins D, Harcourt-Webster JN, et al. Oesophageal symptoms, their causes, treatment and prognosis in patients with the acquired immunodeficiency syndromes. Gut 30:1033-1039, 1989.

4. Eisner MS, Smith PD. Etiology of odynophagia and dysphagia in patients with AIDS. Gastroenterology 98:A446, 1990.

5. Bonacini M, Young T, Laine L. The causes of esophageal symptoms in human immunodeficiency virus infection. A prospective study of 110 patients. Arch Intern Med 151:1567-1572, 1991.

6. Raufman J-P, Tavitian A, Straus EW. Diagnostic, therapeutic and prognostic implications of oral candidiasis in patients with AIDS or AIDS-related complex. Dig Dis Sci 31:476S, 1986.

7. Wilcox CM, Schwartz DA. Etiology, response to therapy and long-term outcome of esophageal ulcer in HIV-infected patients. Gastroenterology 104:A801, 1993.

8. Parente F, Cernuschi M, Rizzardini G, et al. Opportunistic infections of the esophagus not responding to oral systemic antifungals in patients with AIDS: Their frequency and treatment. Am J Gastroenterol 86:1729-1734, 1991.

9. Coleman DC, Bennett DE, Sullivan DJ, et al. Oral *Candida* in HIV infection and AIDS: New perspective/new approaches. Crit Rev Microbiol 19:61-82, 1993.

10. Forsmark CE, Wilcox CM, Darragh T, et al. Disseminated histoplasmosis in AIDS: An unusual case of esophageal involvement and gastrointestinal bleeding. Gastrointest Endosc 36:604-605, 1990.

11. Cappell MS, Armenian BP. Esophagitis from *Candida* or exophiala? Ann Intern Med 115:69, 1991.

12. Wilcox M, Diehl DL, Cello JP, et al. Cytomegalovirus esophagitis in patients with AIDS. A clinical, endoscopic and pathological correlation. Ann Intern Med 113:589-593, 1990.

13. Kitchen VS, Helbert M, Francis ND, et al. Epstein-Barr virus associated oesophageal ulcers in AIDS. Gut 31:1223-1225, 1990.

14. Bartelsman JF, Lange JM, van Leeuwen R, et al. Acute primary HIV-esophagitis. Endoscopy 22:184-185, 1990.

15. Rabeneck L, Popovic M, Gartner S, et al. Acute HIV infection presenting with painful swallowing and esophageal ulcers. JAMA 263:2318-2322, 1990.

16. Ezell JH, Bremer J, Adamec TA. Bacterial esophagitis: An often forgotten cause of odynophagia. Am J Gastroenterol 85:296-298, 1990.

17. de Silva R, Stoopack PM, Raufman JP. Esophageal fistulas associated with mycobacterial infection in patients at risk for AIDS. Radiology 175:449-453, 1990.

18. Allen CM, Craze J, Grundy A. Tuberculosis bronchooesophageal fistula in the acquired immunodeficiency syndrome. Clin Radiol 43:60-62, 1991.

19. Kazlow PG, Shah K, Benkov KJ, et al. Esophageal cryptosporidiosis in a child with acquired immunodeficiency syndrome. Gastroenterology 91:1301-1303, 1986.

20. Grimes MM, LaPook JD, Bar MH, et al. Disseminated *Pneumocystis carinii* infection in a patient with acquired immunodeficiency syndrome. Hum Pathol 18:307-308, 1987.

21. Kotler DP, Reka S, Orenstein JM, et al. Chronic idiopathic esophageal ulceration in the acquired immunodeficiency syndrome. J Clin Gastroenterol 15:284-290, 1992.

22. Wilcox CM. Esophageal diseases in the acquired immunodeficiency syndrome: Etiology, diagnosis and management. Am J Med 92:412-421, 1992.

23. Parente F, Cernuschi M, Valsecchi L, et al. Acute upper gastrointestinal bleeding in patients with AIDS: A relatively uncommon condition associated with reduced survival. Gut 32:987-990, 1991.

24. Cronstedt JL, Bouchama A, Hainau B, et al. Spontaneous esophageal perforation in herpes simplex esophagitis. Am J Gastroenterol 87:124-127, 1992.

25. Bianchi Porro G, Parente F, Cernuschi M. The diagnosis of esophageal candidiasis in patients with the acquired immune deficiency syndrome: Is endoscopy always necessary? Am J Gastroenterol 84:143-146, 1989.

26. Wall SD. Gastrointestinal imaging in AIDS—Luminal gastrointestinal tract. Gastroenterol Clin North Am 17:523-533, 1988.

27. Connolly GM, Forbes A, Gleeson JA, et al. Investigation of upper gastrointestinal symptoms in patients with AIDS. AIDS 3:453-456, 1989.

28. Hanson PJ, Dor G, Jeffries DJ, et al. Elimination of high titre HIV from fiberoptic endoscopes. Gut 31:657-659, 1990.

29. Kodsi BE, Wickremesinghe PC, Kozinn PJ, et al. *Candida* esophagitis: A prospective study of 27 cases. Gastroenterology 71:715-719, 1976.

30. Theise HD, Rotterdam H, Dieterich D. Cytomegalovirus esophagitis in AIDS: Diagnosis by endoscopic biopsy. Am J Gastroenterol 86:1123-1126, 1991.

31. McBane RD, Gross JB. Herpes esophagitis: Clinical syndrome, endoscopic appearance and diagnosis in 23 patients. Gastrointest Endosc 37:600-603, 1991.

32. Bonacini M, Laine L, Gal AA, et al. Prospective evaluation of blind brushings of the esophagus for *Candida* esophagitis in patients with human immunodeficiency virus infection. Am J Gastroenterol 85:385-389, 1990.

33. Lalor E, Rabeneck L. Esophageal candidiasis in AIDS. Successful therapy with clotrimazole vaginal tablets taken by mouth. Dig Dis Sci 36:279-281, 1991.

34. Deschamps M-MH, Paper JW, Verdier RI, et al. Treatment of *Candida* esophagitis in AIDS patients. Am J Gastroenterol 83:20-21, 1988.

35. Laine L, Dretler RH, Conteas CN, et al. Fluconazole compared with ketoconazole for the treatment of *Candida* esophagitis in AIDS: A randomized trial. Ann Intern Med 117:655-660, 1992.

36. Smith DE, Midgley J, Allan M, et al. Itraconazole versus ketoconazole in the treatment of oral and oesophageal cardiosis in patients with infected HIV. AIDS 5:1367-1371, 1991.

37. Parente F, Ardizzone S, Cernuschi M, et al. Prevention of symptomatic recurrences of esophageal candidiasis in AIDS patients after the first episode: A prospective open study. Am J Gastroenterol 89:416-420, 1994.

38. Pace F, Parente F, Bianchi Porro G. Nonreflux-related inflammatory esophageal conditions. Curr Opin Gastroenterol 9:649-653, 1993.

39. Blanshard C. Treatment of HIV-related cytomegalovirus disease of the gastrointestinal track with foscarnet. J Acquir Immune Defic Syndr 5 (Suppl):S25-S28, 1992.

40. Dieterich DT, Poles MA, Dicker M, et al. Foscarnet treatment for cytomegalovirus gastrointestinal infection in acquired immunodeficiency patients who have failed ganciclovir induction. Am J Gastroenterol 88:542-547, 1993.

41. Parente F, Bianchi Porro G, and the Foscarnet Italian GI Study Group. Treatment of CMV esophagitis in AIDS patients. A randomized controlled study of foscarnet versus ganciclovir. 1995 (in press).

42. Shortsleeve MJ, Levine MS. Herpes esophagitis in otherwise healthy patients: Clinical and radiographic findings. Radiology 182:859-861, 1992.

43. Wilcox CM, Karowe MW. Esophageal infections: Etiology, diagnosis and management. Gastroenterologist 2:188-206, 1994.

44. Zamost BJ, Hirschberg J, Ippoliti AF, et al. Esophagitis in scleroderma—Prevalence and risk factors. Gastroenterology 97:421-428, 1987.

45. Trier JS, Bjorkman DJ. Esophageal, gastric and intestinal candidiasis. Am J Med 77:39-43, 1984.

46. Mokoena T, Shama DM, Ngakane H, et al. Oesophageal tuberculosis: A review of eleven cases. Postgrad Med J 68:110-115, 1992.

47. Frick T, Fryd DS, Goodale RL, et al. Incidence and treatment of *Candida* oesophagitis in patients undergoing renal transplantation. Am J Surg 155:311-313, 1988.

48. Alexander JA, Brouillette DE, Chien MC, et al. Infectious esophagitis following liver and renal transplantation. Dig Dis Sci 33:1121-1126, 1988.

49. Goodrich JM, Bowden RA, Fisher L, et al. Ganciclovir prophylaxis to prevent cytomegalovirus disease after allogenic marrow transplant. Ann Intern Med 118:173-178, 1993.

7

Laparoscopic Myotomy and Anterior Fundoplication for Achalasia

Luigi Bonavina, M.D. • *Riccardo Rosati, M.D.*
Andrea Segalin, M.D. • *Alberto Peracchia, M.D.*

The aim of treatment of esophageal achalasia is to improve symptoms and restore the transit of saliva and food by reducing the resistance of the lower esophageal sphincter (LES). At present, such an end point can only be reached with pneumatic dilation or with extramucosal myotomy. Proponents of the endoscopic treatment have emphasized that the dilation does not require general anesthesia and can be performed on an outpatient basis, with a quick recovery.[1] However, the recent development of minimally invasive surgery has renewed the interest in the surgical therapy of achalasia.[2] Today, esophageal myotomy is feasible through the thoracoscopic or the laparoscopic approach and is gaining favor as the initial treatment of choice of the disease. Because of the ease of including an antireflux procedure, the laparoscopic approach is becoming increasingly popular.

Since the laparoscopic esophageal myotomy can be hazardous because of the loss of tactile perception, we have devised a technique that allows gentle distention of the esophagogastric junction using a balloon dilator inserted in the esophageal lumen through the operating channel of a video endoscope.[3,4] The endoscope is helpful in the identification of the esophagogastric junction, in the performance of the myotomy, and to control its completeness. The technique and the early results of the laparoscopic Heller-Dor procedure are presented.

PATIENTS AND METHODS

From January 1992 to December 1994, a laparoscopic treatment of esophageal achalasia was attempted in 36 patients. There were 19 men and 17 women, with a mean age of 40 years (range, 14 to 65 years). Seven patients had previously undergone one or more unsuccessful sessions of pneumatic dilation of the cardia. Preoperative workup included a barium swallow study, esophagoscopy, and esophageal manometry. Patient follow-up consisted of a clinical and radiographic evaluation 1 to 2 months after surgery and esophageal manometry within the first year postoperatively. Subsequent outpatient visits were scheduled every year.

SURGICAL TECHNIQUE

The laparoscopic approach must fulfill some important technical principles that have been used in open surgery for several years[5]: minimal dissection of the hiatal attachments; complete division of the longitudinal and circular muscle fibers for at least 6 cm of the esophagus; extension of the myotomy for at least 2 cm onto the stomach; construction of a partial fundoplication to prevent gastroesophageal reflux; and healing of the edges of the myotomy.

The patient is placed on the operating table in a 20- to 30-degree reverse Trendelenburg lithotomy position. The surgeon stands between the patient's legs. Once the pneumoperitoneum is established, the abdominal cavity is entered through a 10 mm disposable trocar placed in the left upper quadrant approximately at the level of the midclavicular line (initially for the scope, then used as an operating port). Four additional ports are then placed under direct vision: (1) a 10 mm trocar in the midline 4 to 5 cm above the umbilicus (scope); (2) a 10 mm trocar in the right hypochondrium (liver retraction); (3) a 5 mm trocar in the midline just below the xiphoid (grasping and dissecting); and (4) a 5 mm trocar in the left upper quadrant along the axillary line (stomach grasping and retraction). Either a direct or a 30-degree scope can be used. Although the angled scope can provide a better view of the hiatal region, the direct scope has always proved suitable in our experience. After trocar placement, an esophagoscope is introduced in the esophageal lumen and a guidewire is advanced through the operating channel into the stomach.

After incision of the phrenoesophageal membrane, dissection is limited to the anterior aspect of the esophagus and the superior part of diaphragmatic crura. Care is taken not to injure the anterior vagus nerve and its hepatic branch. A low-compliance 30 mm balloon dilator (Rigiflex; Microvasive, Watertown, Mass.) is introduced under endoscopic control over the wire and positioned at the esophagogastric junction. The correct position of the balloon is checked by placing the endoscope 2 to 3 cm above the cranial margin of the dilator. A gentle inflation of the balloon, keeping a pressure of less than 1 psi, allows mild distention of the lower esophagus and cardia. Myotomy is begun with the hook on the anterior aspect of the distal esophagus. The muscle fibers are divided and the submucosal plane is reached. Bleeding is minimal, so coagulation should be used at a very low voltage. By lifting the right edge of the myotomy, the muscular layer is dissected from the submucosa and the myotomy is extended cranially for approximately 6 cm. This maneuver is performed using gentle curved endoscopic scissors. Alternate inflation and deflation of the dilator are useful to dissect free the anterior hemicircumference of the submucosa, to divide all residual circular muscular fibers that are easily identified by balloon distention, and to provide transillumination through the endoscope. The myotomy is extended caudally with the hook for 2 cm below the cardia and is directed toward the left anterolateral aspect of the esophagogastric junction, which helps in the identification of the proximal oblique muscular fibers of the stomach, which must be transected. After completion of the myotomy and removal of the dilator, video endoscopy is performed to check for completeness of the myotomy and for mucosal integrity.

The anterior fundoplication is then constructed. The anterior fundic wall is sutured first to the left and then to the right muscular edge of the myotomy with three interrupted stitches for each side (2-0 Ti-Cron for intracorporeal and 3-0 Prolene for extracorporeal knotting). The proximal suture of the right side also includes the superior part of the right crus. A nasogastric tube is left in place until the second postoperative day and removed after a Gastrografin swallow study has shown a good esophageal transit and no evidence of leaks.

RESULTS

Based on radiographic criteria, patients were classified as having grade I (n = 7), grade II (n = 25), or grade III (n = 4) achalasia. There were three conversions to laparotomy. In two patients there was a mucosal tear, which occurred in one patient because of hypertrophy of the left lobe of the liver that made exposure of the hiatus difficult.

In the remaining 33 patients, the mean duration of the laparoscopic procedure was 140 minutes. There was no operative mortality. A mucosal tear was promptly repaired with fine sutures and did not require conversion in three patients who had previously undergone pneumatic dilations of the cardia.

The postoperative course was uneventful in all but one patient in whom a hemorrhage from a stress gastric ulcer occurred. The Gastrografin swallow study, performed on the second postoperative day in all but three patients, showed satisfactory esophageal emptying and the reappearance of the gastric air pocket. In the three patients with a mucosal tear, the radiographic study was postponed to the seventh postoperative day and was normal.

The clinical result of the operation was satisfactory in all but one patient. At a mean follow-up time of 13 months (range, 3 to 27 months), the only patient with recurrent dysphagia was successfully treated by pneumatic dilation of the cardia.

Postoperative barium swallow study 1 to 2 months after surgery showed a reduction of the mean diameter of the esophageal lumen from 49 to 29 mm. Esophageal manometry was performed in 20 patients 1 to 12 months after the operation. The LES tone decreased from 31 to 12 mm Hg and the LES residual pressure decreased from 15 to 4 mm Hg. It is of interest to note that mean postoperative LES tone obtained with the laparoscopic procedure is comparable to that obtained after open surgery in our institution.

DISCUSSION

The transabdominal esophageal myotomy combined with an anterior fundoplication is one of the most commonly performed procedures for the treatment of esophageal achalasia. The long-term results of this operation have shown relief of dysphagia in over 90% of patients and a less than 10% incidence of postoperative gastroesophageal reflux.[5-8]

As soon as the advantages of laparoscopic surgery in terms of postoperative comfort and patient satisfaction became evident, we decided to apply the same principles of open surgery to the minimally invasive approach. However, esophageal myotomy is more difficult to perform laparoscopically because of the absence of tactile perception. This may lead to an increased risk of incomplete myotomy and mucosal tear. In an attempt to make the procedure safer, we devised a new method, the intraoperative balloon distention of the esophagogastric junction, to ease the myotomy.

As it was our policy in open surgery, dissection of the cardia is limited to the anterior aspect of the esophagogastric junction because we consider the preservation of the anatomic relationships to be of the utmost importance to prevent postoperative gastroesophageal reflux. Endoscopy and balloon distention allow identification and division of the residual circular muscle fibers after myotomy is performed. The distention of the cardia decreases the amount of bleeding, thus the need for electrocoagulation, which is always hazardous at this time, is minimized.

A crucial point in the technique is the extension of the myotomy onto the stomach. Incompleteness of the myotomy at this site leads to persistent or recurrent achalasia. Technically, this is the most demanding part of the operation. The hook is the most suitable instrument to divide the muscle component of the anterior gastric wall. The changing direction of the muscular fibers, from circular in the esophagus to oblique at the cardia, can better be visualized following esophagoscopic transillumination and mild pneumatic distention of the cardia. Bleeding is also more pronounced at this point of the operation and coagulation must be effective. The addition of a Dor fundoplication provides further protection against postoperative reflux. Moreover, the wrap helps in the prevention of reapproximation of the muscular edges of the myotomy, which could result in late symptomatic recurrence.[9]

An interesting finding in this study is that the laparoscopic Heller-Dor operation gives similar functional results compared to the open procedure. The fact that the mean postoperative resting pressures of the LES are comparable indicates that the same technical principles have been applied and the same physiologic changes have been induced using the two surgical methods.

CONCLUSION

Minimally invasive surgery has added a new dimension to the treatment of achalasia. The laparoscopic myotomy combined with a Dor fundoplication is feasible and safe, provided that the same technical principles already applied in open surgery are closely observed. Conversion to laparotomy must be considered if exposure is difficult or if a large mucosal perforation occurs. Intraoperative balloon distention of the cardia may facilitate the procedure and increase its safety.

The preliminary clinical and functional results show the effectiveness of this operation. The main advantages of the laparoscopic approach over the open procedure are the excellent view of the operative field because of the magnifying effect of the telescopic camera and the reduced operative trauma leading to increased patient acceptance of the operation. Laparoscopic surgery may therefore become the first option in the treatment of esophageal achalasia because it offers comparable results to the open approach with minimal morbidity and discomfort.

REFERENCES

1. Cusumano A, Bonavina L, Norberto L, et al. Early and long-term results of pneumatic dilation in the treatment of oesophageal achalasia. Surg Endosc 5:9, 1991.
2. Peracchia A, Ancona E, Ruol A, et al. Use of mini-invasive procedures in esophageal surgery. Chirurgie 118:305-309, 1992.
3. Ancona E, Peracchia A, Zaninotto G, et al. Heller laparoscopic cardiomyotomy with antireflux anterior fundoplication (Dor) in the treatment of esophageal achalasia. Surg Endosc 7:459-461, 1993.
4. Rosati R, Fumagalli U, Bonavina L, et al. Laparoscopic approach to esophageal achalasia. Am J Surg 169:424-427, 1995.
5. Bonavina L, Nosadini A, Bardini R, et al. Primary treatment of esophageal achalasia. Long-term results of myotomy and Dor fundoplication. Arch Surg 127:222-226, 1992.
6. Csendes A, Braghetto I, Mascaro J, et al. Late subjective and objective evaluation of the results of esophagomyotomy in 100 patients with achalasia of the esophagus. Surgery 104:469-475, 1988.
7. Desa L, Spencer J, McPherson S. Surgery for achalasia cardiae: The Dor operation. Ann R Coll Surg Engl 72:128-131, 1990.
8. Gerzic Z, Knezevic J, Milicevic M, et al. Results of transabdominal cardiomyotomy with Dor partial fundoplication in the management of achalasia. In Siewert JR, Holscher AH, eds. Diseases of the Esophagus. Berlin: Springer-Verlag, 1988, pp 970-974.
9. Peracchia A, Bonavina L, Nosadini A, et al. Management of recurrent symptoms after esophagomyotomy for achalasia. Dis Esoph 3:25-28, 1990.

8

Thoracoscopic Myotomy

Peter F. Crookes, M.D. • *Jeffrey H. Peters*, M.D. • *Tom R. DeMeester*, M.D.

The characteristic abnormality in esophageal motor disorders is the presence of deranged transport of a bolus from the esophagus into the stomach in the absence of a mechanically obstructing lesion or the presence of spontaneous contractile activity. The purpose of surgery in esophageal motor disorders is to relieve the outflow obstruction imposed by a nonrelaxing lower esophageal sphincter (LES), to abolish simultaneous contractions in the esophageal body, or to resect an esophageal diverticulum that has developed in response to the motor disorder. The decision to offer surgical treatment for motor disorders is complex and requires a thorough understanding of their pathophysiology.

Patients commonly present with dysphagia, chest pain, regurgitation, or pulmonary symptoms. Depending on which symptom is dominant, the cause may be wrongly attributed to cardiac, gastric, or pulmonary disease. If no such cause is detected on initial investigation, the patient may be dismissed with a diagnosis of anxiety or stress-related disorder. Many of these elementary mistakes may be avoided by taking a careful and detailed history. Subsequent investigation is directed toward excluding a structural cause by barium radiography and endoscopy and defining the nature and extent of the physiologic dysfunction by manometric studies.

Dysphagia is the primary symptom of esophageal motor disorders. Its perception by the patient is a balance between the severity of the underlying abnormality and the adjustment made by the patient in altering his or her eating habits. Because the adjustment is initially unconscious, detailed questioning is required to uncover its extent (e.g., whether the patient requires liquids with the meal, limits the type of food eaten, cuts food into small pieces, is the last to finish, interrupts a meal to regurgitate, or has been admitted to the hospital for food impaction). It is also important to distinguish vomiting from regurgitation because the patient may mislead the clinician by describing the regurgitation of bland-tasting recently ingested food as vomiting. In addition, a history of weight loss should be sought. These assessments help to quantitate the dysphagia and provide a measure of the extent to which the disorder has interfered with the patient's physical and social health. They are also important in determining the indications for, and assessing the outcome of, surgical therapy.

Patients whose primary symptom is chest pain are usually referred only after cardiac evaluation has excluded organic heart disease. An esophageal source is usually only considered when the chest pain accompanies eating or if dysphagia is present. Because dysphagia causes subconscious adaptation in eating habits, it may not be volunteered by the patient unless specifically questioned. Occasionally, primary motor disorders cause primary respiratory complaints such as nocturnal choking and aspiration, but these symptoms tend to be common in advanced disease when the diagnosis is more obvious.

Table 8-1 Current classification of esophageal motility disorders

Primary esophageal motility disorders	Secondary esophageal motility disorders
Achalasia, "vigorous" achalasia	Collagen vascular diseases: Progressive systemic
Diffuse and segmental esophageal spasm	sclerosis, polymyositis and dermatomyositis,
Nutcracker esophagus	mixed connective tissue disease, systemic lupus
Hypertensive lower esophageal sphincter	erythematosis, etc.
Nonspecific esophageal motility disorders	Chronic idiopathic intestinal pseudo-obstruction
	Neuromuscular diseases
	Endocrine and metastatic disorders

Table 8-2 Characteristics of the primary esophageal motility disorders on standard manometry

Achalasia

Incomplete lower esophageal sphincter relaxation (<75% relaxation)
Aperistalsis in the esophageal body
Elevated lower esophageal sphincter pressure (>26 mm Hg)
Increased intraesophageal baseline pressures relative to gastric baseline

Diffuse esophageal spasm

Simultaneous (nonperistaltic contractions) (>20% of wet swallows)
Intermittent normal peristalsis
Repetitive and multipeaked contractions
Spontaneous contractions
Contractions of increased amplitude and duration

Nutcracker esophagus

Mean peristaltic amplitude in the distal esophagus >180 mm Hg
Normal peristaltic sequence

Hypertensive lower esophageal sphincter

Elevated lower esophageal sphincter resting pressure (>26 mm Hg)
Normal lower esophageal sphincter relaxation
Normal peristalsis in the esophageal body

Nonspecific esophageal motility disorders

Decreased or absent amplitude of esophageal peristalsis
Increased number of nontransmitted contractions
Abnormal waveforms
Normal mean lower esophageal sphincter pressure and relaxation

CLASSIFICATION OF ESOPHAGEAL MOTOR DISORDERS

Esophageal motor disorders are classified as either primary or secondary.[1] The cause of the underlying defect in primary motor disorders is not known. There are four named categories of primary esophageal motor disorders: (1) achalasia, (2) diffuse esophageal spasm, (3) nutcracker esophagus, and (4) hypertensive LES. A fifth category, nonspecific esophageal motor disorder (NEMD), is used to describe patients whose motility patterns are clearly outside the normal range, but do not fit into one of the specific categories (Table 8-1). This classification is based on the assessment of 10 wet swallows during stationary manometry (Table 8-2). The more physiologic technique of ambulatory manometry assesses about 100 times as many waves under a variety of physiologic conditions and may in the future be able to classify motor disorders more clearly.[2,3] Secondary motor disorders are caused by an underlying connective tissue or muscle disease affecting the esophagus, such as scleroderma or dermatomyositis. The clinical and manometric features of these disorders are described in Chapter 1. This chapter describes only those features relevant to surgery.

ACHALASIA

Achalasia is the best known primary motility disorder of the esophagus. It is characterized by failure of esophageal body peristalsis and incomplete relaxation of the LES (Fig. 8-1). It is generally thought to be caused by neuronal degeneration

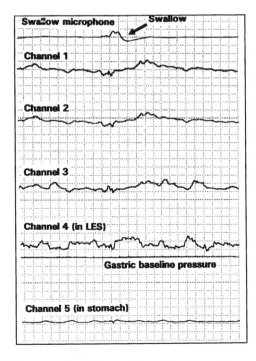

Fig. 8-1   Motility record demonstrating failure of the sphincter to relax on swallowing and elevation of intraluminal esophageal pressure and aperistalsis in the body of the esophagus.

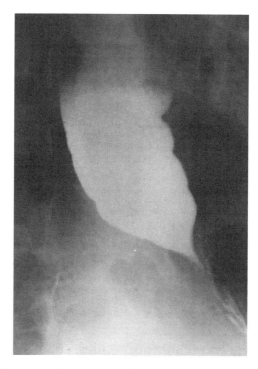

Fig. 8-2 Barium esophagogram showing a markedly dilated esophagus and characteristic "bird's beak" in achalasia. (From Waters PF, DeMeester TR. Foregut motor disorders and their surgical treatment. Med Clin North Am 65:1244, 1981.)

in the myenteric plexus of the esophageal wall, causing aperistalsis, and loss of activity of inhibitory neurons in the LES leading to incomplete LES relaxation. The cause of the neuronal degeneration is obscure. There is some evidence that previous infection with varicella-zoster virus may be responsible. In experimental animals, the disease has been reproduced by destruction of the nucleus ambiguus and the dorsal motor nucleus of the vagus. However, there is some experimental evidence that incomplete obstruction at the gastroesophageal junction may produce a condition with the radiologic and manometric features of achalasia.[4] This corresponds to the clinical situation where features of achalasia develop in response to an infiltrating tumor of the cardia (pseudoachalasia) or after a tight Nissen fundoplication or Angelchick prosthesis. This evidence suggests that loss of LES relaxation is a primary phenomenon and the degeneration of the esophageal body is secondary. The corollary to this view is that early diagnosis and definitive treatment is important in limiting or even reversing esophageal body deterioration.

Regardless of the initiating factor, the combination of a nonrelaxing sphincter, which causes a functional holdup of ingested material in the esophagus, and elevation of intraluminal pressure from repetitive pharyngeal swallowing results in dilation of the esophageal body. With time, the functional disorder results in anatomic alterations that are seen on radiographic studies as a dilated esophagus with a tapering, beak-like narrowing of the distal end (Fig. 8-2). There is usually an air fluid

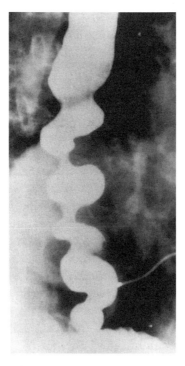

Fig. 8-3   Barium esophagogram of patient with diffuse esophageal spasm showing the "corkscrew" deformity.

level in the esophagus, the height of which reflects the resistance imposed by the nonrelaxing sphincter. A hazy pattern within the esophagus suggests retained food particles. As the disease progresses, the esophagus becomes greatly dilated and tortuous.

A subgroup of patients with otherwise typical features of classic achalasia have simultaneous contractions of the esophageal body that can be of high amplitude. This manometric pattern has been termed "vigorous achalasia" and chest pain episodes are a common finding in these patients. Differentiation of vigorous achalasia from diffuse esophageal spasm can be difficult. In both diseases barium studies may show a corkscrew deformity of the esophagus and diverticulum formation (Fig. 8-3).

Treatment Options

It is generally agreed that drug treatment of achalasia is ineffective. The only treatments in widespread use are surgical myotomy, balloon dilation, and more recently, botulinum toxin injection. All treatments aim to reduce outflow resistance by dividing, stretching, or paralyzing the LES. The most novel treatment, injection of the LES with botulinum toxin via the flexible endoscope, is an attractive option in that it is truly minimally invasive and of low cost, but the published results are of very small series of patients followed up for short periods of time.[5] Thus its ultimate role remains to be evaluated. The mainstay of treatment for achalasia is therefore either surgical myotomy or balloon dilation. Only one randomized trial has compared myotomy with dilation and this showed a clear advantage for surgery.[6] This trial was criticized because the dilations were not performed in what is now the standard manner. However, there are several nonrandomized comparisons in the literature, all of which come to the same conclusion.[7,8] Balloon dilation has the advantage because it is performed on an outpatient basis and requires no general anesthetic. Its cost is therefore low. However, there is a substantial risk of perforation (5% to 8%). When perforation does occur, it may respond well to nonoperative therapy, but if a subsequent myotomy is necessary, the fibrosis surrounding the healed perforation makes the procedure much more difficult. The chief advantage of myotomy is a more uniform relief of dysphagia because of the more exact disruption of the LES. This is especially true in younger patients, many of whom respond poorly to dilation. Any form of treatment that reduces LES resistance sufficiently to provide relief of dysphagia may increase the risk of pathologic gastroesophageal reflux. The long-term incidence of gastroesophageal reflux after myotomy is probably higher than after dilation, but comparative studies with 24-hour esophageal pH monitoring are lacking.[9]

Myotomy of the LES is recommended as the primary treatment of achalasia unless the patient is very elderly or suffers from serious comorbid illness making administration of a general anesthetic hazardous.

Myotomy of the Lower Esophageal Sphincter

Four important principles are followed when surgical myotomy of the LES is performed: (1) minimal dissection of the cardia, (2) adequate distal myotomy to reduce outflow resistance, (3) prevention of postoperative reflux, and (4) prevention of rehealing of the myotomy site. These principles are followed regardless of whether the myotomy is performed thoracoscopically, by open transthoracic route, or through the abdomen. From a practical standpoint, there are two major controversies, specifically, the extent of the myotomy and whether to add an antireflux procedure.

The proximal limit is determined by the manometric findings. In typical achalasia, where there are no active contractions in the esophageal body, the myotomy extends proximally to just above the LES, approximately 6 cm above the gastroesophageal junction. If simultaneous esophageal contractions are associated with the sphincter abnormality, so-called vigorous achalasia, the myotomy should extend over the distance of the motility abnormality as mapped by the preoperative motility study. Failure to do this may result in continuing dysphagia and a dissatisfied patient.

The distal extent of the myotomy and the addition of an antireflux procedure are closely related issues and to some extent depend on the surgeon's philosophy. Some surgeons, to be sure that the myotomy is adequate, extend it well beyond the gastroesophageal junction, recognizing that this may predispose to postoperative gastroesophageal reflux.[10] Those surgeons add an antireflux procedure, usually by a partial fundoplication, which may be either anterior (Dor) or posterior (Toupet).[11,12] Donahue et al.,[13] who developed the so-called "floppy Nissen," recommend a floppy full 360-degree wrap after myotomy. However, the experience of most other surgeons is that a complete 360-degree wrap imposes too great an obstruction for the aperistaltic esophageal body to overcome, and long-term recurrence of dysphagia is likely.[14] In contrast to this view, Ellis, Crozier, and Watkins[15] argue that a myotomy extending only a few millimeters onto the stomach, coupled with minimal dissection of the perihiatal attachments of the cardia, allows a satisfactory compromise between reduction of LES resistance and reflux protection.

These two issues are relevant to thoracoscopic myotomy because definition of the distal extent of the myotomy is enhanced by the magnified thoracoscopic image and aided by simultaneous endoluminal endoscopy. However, the addition of an antireflux procedure is much more difficult than at open myotomy.[16] Consequently, most reports of thoracoscopic myotomy, including our own, have adopted the philosophy of limited myotomy and minimal perihiatal dissection to provide adequate antireflux protection.

Technique

The procedure is performed with the patient in the right lateral decubitus position and with the surgeon standing on the left side of the table facing the patient's back. A double-lumen endotracheal tube is used to allow selective ventilation of the right lung. An assistant is available to pass the flexible upper gastrointestinal endoscope into the esophagus for simultaneous visualization of the myotomy.

Port placement. A four-port technique is employed in addition to a small (1-inch) incision along the left costal margin for placement of retracting instruments (Fig. 8-4). A 10 mm port placed posterior to the scapula in the fourth intercostal space is used for the camera. Meticulous hemostasis is important when the trocar holes are made. Bleeding from the trocar sites is common and very troublesome during the procedure, particularly from the camera port. Air is allowed to enter the thorax and the left lung is slowly deflated, with some assistance from the shaft of the telescope. A second 10 mm port is placed high and anterior in the second or third intercostal space at the anterior axillary line. A Babcock clamp placed through this port is used as a lung retractor following incision of the inferior pulmonary ligament. The surgeon's right-handed port is placed at the midaxillary line in the sixth or seventh intercostal space. The position should be such that the electrocautery hook placed through the right-handed trocar is directly above the esophagus and not approaching it from an angle. If this trocar is placed too high, there may be difficulty in performing the myotomy near the gastroesophageal junction. The surgeon's left-handed trocar is placed low, inferior and posterior, above the diaphragm in the ninth or tenth intercostal space. Finally, a single 2-inch incision is made along the left costal margin directly above the esophagus for placement of three instruments: a fan retractor to displace the diaphragm inferiorly, a long vein retractor to retract the crura superiorly, and a suction irrigation device.

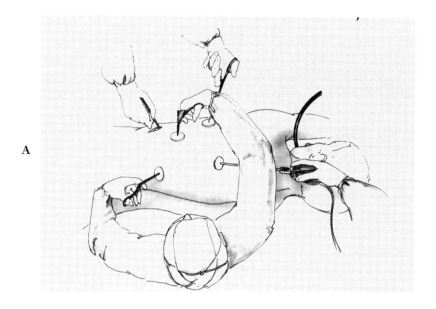

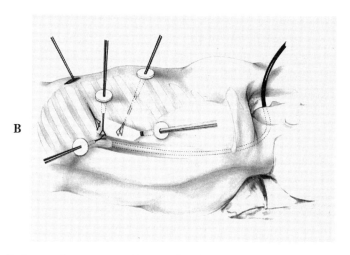

Fig. 8-4 A, Patient and surgeon positioning for thoracoscopic esophageal myotomy. **B,** Trocar placement. Four 10 mm thoracoports and a single 2- to 3-inch incision are used.

With selective ventilation of the right lung, it is not necessary to insufflate the left hemithorax. One of the advantages of thoracoscopy is that air-tight ports are not necessary, thus allowing small incisions and the placement of standard instruments. We have found that a 30-degree telescope is preferable to a 0-degree scope.

Retraction. Proper retraction and exposure of the esophagus and hiatus are critical to the dissection and require some attention at the outset. The diaphragm should be strongly displaced inferiorly using the large fan retractor, thus exposing

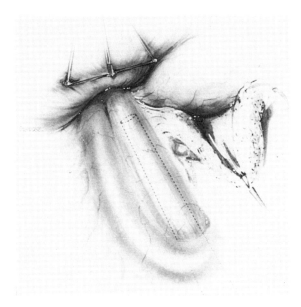

Fig. 8-5 Thoracoscopic esophageal myotomy illustrating the exposure obtained with video-assisted technology. This allows the traditional myotomy of the esophageal lower sphincter or body to be performed without a thoracotomy. The diaphragm is forcefully retracted toward the abdomen with a fan-shaped retractor inserted through a small incision along the left costal border. The left lower lung is retracted superiorly and anteriorly by a Babcock clamp placed in a high anterior port.

the esophageal hiatus. Identification and dissection of the esophagus is aided by the concomitant use of an endoscope within the esophageal lumen, allowing displacement of the esophagus to the left. In patients with achalasia the esophagus is often dilated and easily seen. The mediastinal pleura overlying the terminal esophagus is divided sharply with scissors and the inferior pulmonary ligament divided for 2 to 3 cm. A Babcock clamp placed through the high anterior port is used to retract the left lung toward the superior thorax (Fig. 8-5).

Initial dissection. The dissection is consciously kept to a minimum, preserving normal hiatal structures. The phrenoesophageal membrane is incised, allowing placement of a long vein retractor underneath the crural arch and retraction of the crura away from the esophagus. The gastric serosa usually becomes evident and is recognized by its more distinct white color. No attempt is made to mobilize any portion of the stomach because only visualization of the gastroesophageal junction is necessary (Fig. 8-6).

The myotomy. The myotomy is begun 2 to 3 cm above the gastroesophageal junction and performed with a L-hook electrocautery probe (Fig. 8-7). The magnification of the telescope usually allows clear visualization of the longitudinal and circular muscle fibers. Insufflation through an intraluminal flexible endoscope al-

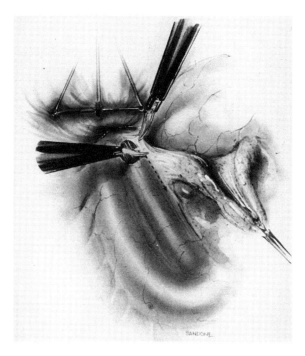

Fig. 8-6 Videoscopic view of the initial dissection for myotomy of the LES. The pleura overlying the lower esophagus is being incised.

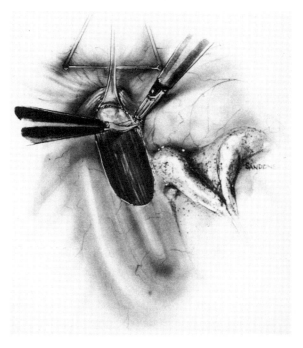

Fig. 8-7 The initial dissection is continued by dissecting the crura of the diaphragm at the gastro-esophageal junction.

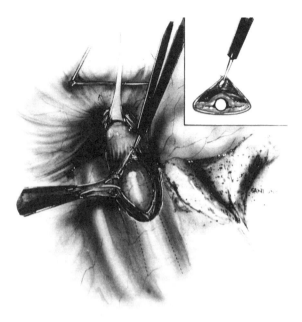

Fig. 8-8   The myotomy is begun 1 to 2 cm above the gastroesophageal junction and carried out with an L-hook electrocautery instrument. Note the intraluminal endoscope is an aid in defining the gastroesophageal junction. The inset demonstrates collapse of the mucosa as suction is applied via the endoscope just prior to the application of electrocautery.

lows the mucosa to pouch out between the cut ends of the muscle, clearly outlining the myotomized segment. In addition, the endoscope within the lumen of the esophagus can be used to help prevent mucosal injury by applying suction to collapse the mucosa prior to using the electrocautery. Once the esophageal mucosa is clearly identified, the myotomy is carried distally with an electrocautery probe or scissors. The inferior extent of the myotomy is carefully judged through the endoscope. The myotomy is discontinued when it has reached the endoscopic gastroesophageal junction and the spasm of the valve commonly associated with achalasia is alleviated (Fig. 8-8).

Closure. At the completion of the procedure the dependent portion of the left chest is filled with water and air is insufflated through the endoscope to check for esophageal mucosal integrity (Fig. 8-9). A small-caliber chest tube is placed and the left lung is reinflated under direct vision. All trocars are removed and the wounds are closed in a two-layer fashion.

Postoperative Care

A nasogastric tube is not necessary. Its placement is potentially hazardous following myotomy. A video contrast esophagogram is performed the day following surgery and, if it is acceptable, the patient is allowed liquids. Hospital stay in the absence of comorbid disease is generally 2 to 3 days.

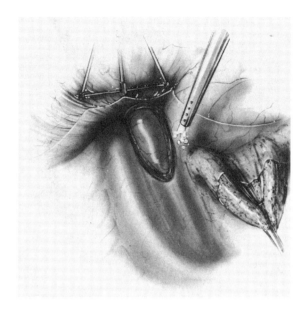

Fig. 8-9 Following completion of the myotomy the lower chest and esophagus are irrigated with water. The integrity of the esophageal mucosa is checked by insufflating air through the intraluminal endoscope.

Results

Critical analysis of the results of therapy for motor disorders of the esophagus requires objective measurement. Almost all patients experience immediate improvement in dysphagia. However, the use of symptoms alone as an end point to evaluate therapy may be misleading. Just as in the initial evaluation, the propensity of patients modifying their diet to avoid difficulty swallowing is often underestimated, making an assessment of results based on symptoms unreliable. Objective evidence early in the postoperative course may indicate the probability of future recurrence of symptoms. A satisfactory decrease in outflow resistance should therefore be included in any careful evaluation of treatment results.

A variety of objective measurements may be used, including reduction in LES pressure, esophageal baseline pressure, and scintigraphic assessment of esophageal emptying time. Of these, the most widely studied is the reduction in LES pressure. Eckardt, Aignherr, and Bernhard[17] recently investigated whether the effect of pneumatic dilation in patients with achalasia could be predicted on the basis of objective measurements. Postdilation LES pressure was the most valuable measurement for predicting long-term clinical response. A postdilation sphincter pressure less than 10 mm Hg predicted a good response. Fifty percent of the patients studied had postdilation sphincter pressures between 10 and 20 mm Hg, with a 2-year remission rate of 71%. They noted that 16 of 46 patients were left with a postdilation sphincter pressure of greater than 20 mm Hg and had an unfavorable outcome.

Open surgery. The study of Csendes et al.[6] showed that myotomy was associated with a significant increase in the diameter at the gastroesophageal junction and a decrease in esophageal body diameter in the midesophagus on follow-up radiographic studies. Further, there was a greater reduction in sphincter pressure and improvement in the amplitude of esophageal contractions following myotomy. Of interest, 13% of patients regained some peristalsis after dilation compared to 28% after surgery. These findings were shown to persist over 5 years of follow-up at which time 95% of those treated with surgical myotomy had a satisfactory outcome. Of those who received dilation, only 54% were doing well, 16% required redilation, and 22% eventually required surgical myotomy to obtain relief.

Bonavina et al.[11] reported good to excellent results with transabdominal myotomy and Dor fundoplication in 94% of patients after a mean follow-up time of 5.4 years. Eighty-one of 193 patients underwent postoperative 24-hour esophageal pH study and only 8.6% of these demonstrated abnormal esophageal acid exposure. Recovery of peristalsis in the esophageal body, as reported by Csendes et al.,[6] was noted in several patients who volunteered for follow-up manometry. This would suggest that the deterioration of esophageal body function in patients with achalasia is secondary to the outflow obstruction of the hypertensive, nonrelaxing LES and is reversible if the obstruction is completely and promptly relieved. Stipa et al.[18] also reported good to excellent long-term results for myotomy in 85% of 101 patients with achalasia after a median follow-up time of approximately 10 years. No operative mortality occurred in either of these series, attesting to the safety of the procedure.

Thoracoscopic myotomy. Early experience with endosurgical esophageal myotomy is encouraging. Pellegrini et al.[16] have reported on 17 patients. Fifteen underwent a thoracoscopic approach and two were approached laparoscopically. Postoperatively, the mean LES pressure was 10 mm Hg, compared with 32 mm Hg preoperatively. Most patients were fed on the second postoperative day, and the average hospital stay was 3 days. There were no deaths or major complications. The relief of dysphagia was graded as excellent in 12 patients, good in two patients, fair in two patients, and poor in one patient.[16] Their subsequent report of 22 patients showed that in the first three patients, the myotomy was incomplete and remyotomy was required. One patient developed a paraesophageal hernia 6 months postoperatively, emphasizing the need for minimal dissection of the cardia.[19]

Our own experience with thoracoscopic myotomy of the LES includes 12 patients. Two patients have required conversion to open surgery. The first patient was converted to inspect the dissection and a second because of a small perforation at the gastroesophageal junction made just after the completion of the myotomy. This was recognized immediately and repaired through a thoracotomy with no postoperative problems. The median age of these patients was 65 years (range, 30 to 83 years). The average duration of thoracoscopic surgery was 223 minutes and the average length of hospitalization was 4 days.

Excellent to good symptomatic results were achieved in the majority of patients (Fig. 8-10). Physiologic studies revealed a significant reduction in mean LES pres-

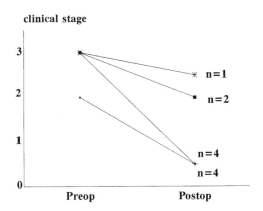

Fig. 8-10 Mean values for the clinical stage of patients before and after thoracoscopic esophageal myotomy.

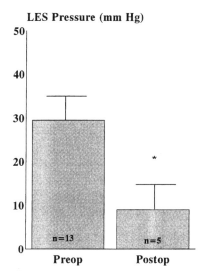

Fig. 8-11 Mean LES pressures before and after thoracoscopic esophageal myotomy. * = p <0.05 vs. preoperatively.

sure (Fig. 8-11) but little change in sphincter length (Fig. 8-12). The manometric effect of myotomy can be illustrated by using three-dimensional reconstructions of the LES[20] (Fig. 8-13). Based on these early results, the symptomatic and objective outcome of thoracoscopic myotomy is equivalent to that of open surgery, and it is associated with the standard advantages of the minimally invasive approach.

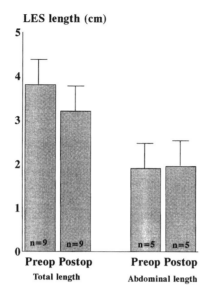

Fig. 8-12   Mean LES total and abdominal lengths before and after thoracoscopic esophageal myotomy.

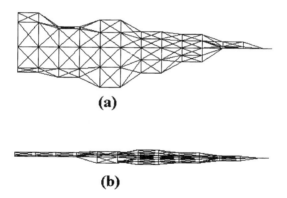

Fig. 8-13   Three-dimensional "wireframe" representation of the LES in a patient with achalasia before treatment **(a)** and after thoracoscopic myotomy **(b)**.

DIFFUSE AND SEGMENTAL ESOPHAGEAL SPASM

This esophageal motor disorder is characterized clinically by substernal chest pain and/or dysphagia. Diffuse esophageal spasm differs from classic achalasia in that it is primarily a disease of the esophageal body, produces a lesser degree of dysphagia, causes more chest pain, and has less effect on the patient's general condition. True diffuse esophageal spasm is a rare condition, occurring approximately five times less frequently than achalasia.

The etiology and neuromuscular pathophysiology of diffuse esophageal spasm are unclear. The basic motor abnormality is rapid progression of contractions down the esophagus secondary to an abnormality in the latency gradient. Hypertrophy of the muscular layer of the esophageal wall and degeneration of the esophageal branches of the vagus nerve have been observed in this disease, although the latter is not a constant finding.[21,22] Manometric abnormalities in diffuse esophageal spasm may be present in the total length of the esophageal body, but are usually confined to the distal two thirds. In segmental esophageal spasm the manometric abnormalities are confined to a short segment of the esophagus.

The classic manometric finding in these patients is the frequent occurrence of simultaneous and repetitive esophageal contractions that may be of abnormally high amplitude or long duration. Key to the diagnosis of diffuse esophageal spasm is that the esophagus must retain a degree of peristaltic performance in contrast to that seen in achalasia. A criterion of 20% or more simultaneous contractions in 10 wet swallows has been used to diagnose diffuse esophageal spasm.[23] This figure is arbitrary and often debated. A different approach to the identification of a patient with diffuse esophageal spasm, based on the more physiologic ambulatory manometry, has recently been proposed.[2] Discriminate analysis has identified a series of abnormalities on the ambulatory motility record of patients with classic diffuse esophageal spasm. A composite score based on these parameters of the ambulatory motility record has allowed diagnosis of the disease with a sensitivity of 90% and a specificity of 100%. When applied prospectively, this scoring system identified severely deteriorated esophageal motor function in symptomatic patients despite the absence of the classic motility abnormalities of diffuse spasm on standard manometry.

The LES in patients with the disease usually shows normal resting pressure and relaxation on swallowing. A hypertensive sphincter with poor relaxation may also be present. In patients with advanced disease the radiographic appearance of tertiary contractions appears helical and has been termed "corkscrew esophagus" or "pseudodiverticulosis." Patients with segmental or diffuse esophageal spasm can compartmentalize the esophagus and develop an epiphrenic or midesophageal diverticulum.

Myotomy of the Esophageal Body

A long esophageal myotomy is indicated for dysphagia caused by any motor disorder characterized by segmental or generalized simultaneous contractions in a patient whose symptoms are not relieved by medical therapy. Such disorders include diffuse and segmental esophageal spasm, vigorous achalasia, and nonspecific motility disorders associated with a mid- or epiphrenic esophageal diverticulum. The recent introduction of 24-hour ambulatory motility monitoring has greatly aided the identification of patients with symptoms of dysphagia and chest pain who might benefit from a surgical myotomy.

The decision to operate rests on a balance of the patient's symptoms, diet, lifestyle adjustments, and nutritional status, with the driving force being the opportunity to improve the patient's swallowing disability. A long myotomy will abolish the simultaneous waves, leading to an improvement if these waves were responsible for the chest pain and dysphagia. However, the myotomy will also abolish the beneficial peristaltic waves, and therefore also carries the risk of increasing the dysphagia. If ambulatory motility monitoring shows that more than 70% of the waves are simultaneous, the loss of the few remaining peristaltic waves is likely to be counterbalanced by the beneficial abolition of simultaneous waves. This shifts the balance in favor of myotomy.[24] Patients whose only symptom is chest pain do not often have a good result after surgical myotomy.

In patients selected for myotomy of the esophageal body, preoperative manometry is essential to determine the proximal extent of the motor abnormality. The myotomy should extend distally across the LES because the resistance of a normal LES may still be too great for the myotomized esophageal body to overcome.

Technique

The technique of long esophageal myotomy is similar to that of myotomy limited to the LES, except that the lung tends to flop over the esophageal body and must be more extensively retracted. Proper positioning of the patient is critical in permitting lung retraction. A prone position is ideal because it allows the left lung to fall forward away from the esophagus. However, if subsequent conversion to thoracotomy becomes necessary, repositioning and redraping are required. We prefer to place the patient in the right lateral decubitus position and then roll the patient 45 degrees toward the prone position. A beanbag and tape are used to secure the patient. The table is rolled the remaining 45 degrees so that the patient ends up in almost a prone position. If thoracotomy becomes necessary, the table can be rolled back to the lateral position so that access can be performed without difficulty. Prone positioning is the key element, allowing simple retraction of the left lung and thus a long myotomy.

Port placement and the initial dissection are identical to that of a LES myotomy. With suitable lung retraction, the myotomy is performed through all muscle layers, extending distally to the endoscopic gastroesophageal junction and proximally on the esophagus over the distance of the manometric abnormality (Fig. 8-14). The muscle layer is dissected from the mucosa laterally for a distance of 1 cm. Care must be taken to divide all minute muscle bands, particularly in the area of the gastroesophageal junction.

The presence of an epiphrenic diverticulum complicates the thoracoscopic procedure. Dissection of the neck of the diverticulum and division through an endoscopic linear stapler may be possible, but it is often difficult to obtain the correct angle for the stapler, even if it possesses a reticulating device. Once excised, the overlying muscle is closed with interrupted Prolene sutures and the myotomy is performed on the opposite esophageal wall. At present we do not hesitate to convert to open thoracotomy if any difficulty is encountered during excision of an

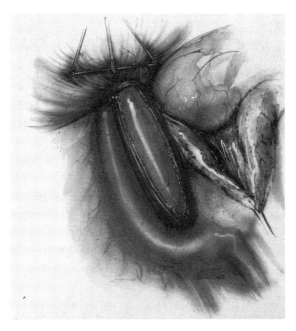

Fig. 8-14   Videoscopic view of long esophageal myotomy at completion of the myotomy.

epiphrenic diverticulum. If a midesophageal diverticulum is present, the myotomy is made so that it includes the neck, following which the diverticulum is inverted and suspended by attaching it to the prevertebral fascia of the thoracic vertebra.

Results

Open long esophageal myotomy. The results of open myotomy for motor disorders of the esophageal body have improved in parallel with the improved preoperative diagnosis afforded by manometry.[25] Previous published series report between 40% and 92% symptomatic improvement, but interpretation is difficult because of the small number of patients involved and the varying criteria for diagnosis of the primary motor abnormality. When this is accurately done, 93% of the patients had effective palliation of dysphagia after a mean follow-up time of 5 years and 89% would have the procedure again if it was necessary. Most patients gain or maintain their weight after the operation. Postoperative motility studies show that myotomy reduces the amplitude of esophageal contractions to near zero, eliminating both simultaneous and peristaltic waves. The dysphagia of the patient is likely to be improved by the procedure only if the benefit of abolishing the simultaneous waves, and as a consequence their adverse effect on bolus propulsion, exceeds the adverse effect on bolus propulsion caused by the loss of the peristaltic waves. If not, the patient is likely to continue to complain of dysphagia and have little improvement from the operation. Thus a delicate balance exists between success and failure of a long esophageal myotomy, which emphasizes the importance of preoperative motility studies.

Thoracoscopic long esophageal myotomy. Preliminary experience with an extended thoracoscopic distal esophageal myotomy for the treatment of nutcracker esophagus has been reported by Cuschieri.[26] Of 23 patients, 18 had a good symptomatic result. No major morbidity was encountered. Nasogastric tubes were removed on the first postoperative day and oral feeding was begun on the second postoperative day. Our own experience includes three such patients, all of whom showed early symptomatic improvement, but who have not yet had postoperative physiologic studies.

CONCLUSION

It is clear that the thoracoscopic treatment of esophageal motor disorders is safe and effective and appears to be comparable to the results of open surgery. Whether long-term follow-up will confirm the early promising results of thoracoscopic procedures remains to be seen and will only be demonstrated by careful and thorough follow-up. Excellent long-term results have been demonstrated with open thoracotomy combining myotomy and partial fundoplication and this should continue to serve as the gold standard for comparison of endosurgical techniques.

Figures 8-4 to 8-12 and 8-14 from Peters JH, DeMeester TR. Thoracoscopic myotomy of the lower esophageal sphincter and esophageal body. In Peters JH, DeMeester TR. Minimally Invasive Surgery of the Foregut. St. Louis: Quality Medical Publishing, 1995, pp 83-102.

REFERENCES

1. DeMeester TR, Stein HJ. Surgery for esophageal motor disorders. In Castell DO, ed. The Esophagus. Boston: Little Brown, 1992, pp 401-439.
2. Eypasch EP, Stein HJ, DeMeester TR, et al. A new technique to define and clarify esophageal motor disorders. Am J Surg 159:144, 1990.
3. Stein HJ, DeMeester TR, Eypasch EP. Ambulatory 24-hour esophageal manometry in the evaluation of esophageal motor disorders and non-cardiac chest pain. Surgery 110:753-763, 1991.
4. Little AG, Correnti FS, Calleja JJ, et al. Effect of incomplete obstruction on feline esophageal function with a clinical correlation. Surgery 100:430, 1986.
5. Pasricha PJ, Ravich WJ, Hendrix TR, et al. Intrasphincteric botulinum toxin for the treatment of achalasia. N Engl J Med 332:774-778, 1995.
6. Csendes A, Braghetto I, Henriquez A, et al. Late results of a prospective randomised study comparing forceful dilatation and oesophagomyotomy in patients with achalasia. Gut 30:299-304, 1989.
7. Okike N, Payne WS. Esophagomyotomy versus forceful dilation for achalasia of the esophagus: Results in 899 patients. Ann Thorac Surg 23:119, 1979.
8. Avranitakis C. Achalasia of the esophagus: A reappraisal of esophagomyotomy vs forceful pneumatic dilatation. Dig Dis 20:841-846, 1975.
9. Andreollo NA, Earlam RJ. Heller's myotomy for achalasia: Is an added antireflux procedure necessary? Br J Surg 74:765-769, 1987.
10. Jara FM, Toledo-Pereya LH, Lewis JW, et al. Long-term results of esophagomyotomy for achalasia of esophagus. Arch Surg 114:935-936, 1979.
11. Bonavina L, Nosadinia A, Bardini R, et al. Primary treatment of esophageal achalasia: Long-term results of myotomy and Dor fundoplication. Arch Surg 127:222-226, 1992.

12. Paricio P, Martinez de Haro L, Ortiz A, et al. Achalasia of the cardia: Long-term results of oesophagomyotomy and posterior partial fundoplication. Br J Surg 77:1371-1374, 1990.
13. Donahue PE, Schlesinger PK, Sluss KF, et al. Esophagocardiomyotomy—Floppy Nissen fundoplication effectively treats achalasia without causing esophageal obstruction. Surgery 116:719-725, 1994.
14. Topart P, Deschamps C, Taillefer R, et al. Long-term effect of total fundoplication on the myotomized esophagus. Ann Thorac Surg 54:1046-1052, 1992.
15. Ellis FH Jr, Crozier RE, Watkins E. The operation for esophageal achalasia: Results of esophagomyotomy without an antireflux operation. J Thorac Cardiovasc Surg 88:344, 1984.
16. Pellegrini C, Wetter LA, Patti M, et al. Thoracoscopic esophagomyotomy. Ann Surg 216:291, 1992.
17. Eckardt VF, Aignherr C, Bernhard G. Predictors of outcome in patients with achalasia treated by pneumatic dilation. Gastroenterology 103:1732-1738, 1992.
18. Stipa S, Fegiz G, Iascone C, et al. Heller-Belsey and Heller-Nissen operations for achalasia of the esophagus. Surg Gynecol Obstet 170:212-216, 1990.
19. Pellegrini C, Leichter R, Patti M, et al. Thoracoscopic esophageal myotomy in the treatment of achalasia. Ann Thorac Surg 56:680-682, 1992.
20. Crookes PF, Heimbucher J, Peters JH, et al. Vector volume analysis demonstrates the effect of treatment of achalasia. Gastroenterology 108:A76, 1995.
21. Ferguson TB, Woodbury JD, Roper CL. Giant muscular hypertrophy of the esophagus. Ann Thorac Surg 8:209, 1969.
22. Gillies M, Nicks R, Skyring A. Clinical, manometric, and pathological studies in diffuse oesophageal spasm. Br Med J 2:527, 1967.
23. Castell DO, Richter JE, Dalton CB, eds. Esophageal Motility Testing. New York: Elsevier, 1987.
24. Eypasch E, DeMeester TR, Klingman R, et al. Physiological assessment and surgical management of diffuse esophageal spasm. J Thorac Cardiovasc Surg 104:859-868, 1992.
25. DeMeester TR. Surgery for esophageal motor disorders. Ann Thorac Surg 34:225, 1982.
26. Cuschieri A. Endoscopic esophageal myotomy for specific motility disorders and non cardiac chest pain. Endosc Surg Allied Technol 1:280-287, 1993.

9

Surgery for Esophageal Diverticula

Ernst Eypasch, M.D. • *Anthony Barlow, F.R.C.S.*

Esophageal diverticula result from an imbalance in the complex and coordinated mechanism of food and saliva transport from the mouth to the stomach. The typical locations are the hypopharyngeal, midesophageal, and epiphrenic areas.

ZENKER'S DIVERTICULUM

Zenker's diverticulum is an outpouching of the posterior pharyngeal mucosa through a weak area called Killian's triangle, which is between the inferior constrictor and the oblique fibers of the cricopharyngeus muscle. Most cases of Zenker's diverticulum develop in the midline and present on the left side of the esophagus.

Different stages in development are stage I, a small barely visible pouch; stage II, a clearly visible diverticulum; and stage III, a large diverticulum that causes displacement of the pharynx with the esophageal orifice upward and to the side.[1,2] Some authors question the clinical relevance of minimal diverticula.[3]

History and Epidemiology

Abraham Ludlow from Bristol was the first to describe a pharyngeal diverticulum and Friedrich Albert Zenker from Munich, whose name became associated with the condition, described a series of 23 cases.[4]

The prevalence of the entity is estimated to be 1 in 1500 individuals.[5] It is the most frequent esophageal outpouching (approximately 70% of all diverticula) and occurs more commonly in the sixth to eighth decades of life.[2]

Anatomy and Physiology

Swallowing, once initiated, is entirely a reflex action. Food, which is taken into the mouth, is propelled by a cylindrical pump action toward the esophagus. The tongue functions as a piston, completely filling the oropharyngeal cylinder and displacing the bolus back into the hypopharynx. This produces a rise in the luminal pressure and causes a pressure gradient between the pharynx and the negative intrathoracic environment. The cricopharyngeal esophageal sphincter relaxes in concert with the pressurization of the pharynx and the bolus of food is literally pulled into the esophagus, moving very rapidly through this region.[6]

The pathogenesis of diverticula is still not completely resolved. Many authors describe functional abnormalities that sound very "logical." Premature contractions, incomplete relaxations, incoordinated intraluminal pressure rises, and functional obstructions have been described, but it is not yet clear whether these phenomena are the cause or the result of the condition.

Proponents of an anatomic explanation stress that the diverticulum is an anatomic abnormality that leads to functional consequences.[3] Because of the fixation of the pharyngeal muscles to the base of the skull and the downward movement of the larynx in erect mammalians, Killian's triangle may vary in size and thus predispose to pouch formation.

Lerut et al.[7] collected morphologic and functional data on the muscles of the cricopharyngeal area and performed functional studies to interpret the clinical results. Operative and autopsy specimens of the cricopharyngeal muscle, the upper esophageal sphincter, and sternocleidomastoid muscle of patients with Zenker's diverticulum were compared to similar specimens from normal controls. Gross pathologic abnormalities could be demonstrated in the musculature of patients, such as changes of fiber type, hypertrophy, atrophy, necrosis, and changes of the cellular muscle structure. Physiologic contractility studies in tubocurarine chloride solutions showed an altered contraction pattern in patients with diverticula. Lerut et al.[7] observed a change from type II fiber (short, fast, forceful contraction) to type I fiber (sustained, tonic, slow, less forceful contraction). However, it is unclear whether this experimentally observed change has a neurogenic or myogenic origin.

Functional and Diagnostic Imaging Studies

Anatomic asymmetries, movement of the pharynx during swallowing, and the inertia of recording systems make manometric evaluation of the cricopharyngeal area difficult and the results controversial.[6] Although the experiments done by Lerut et al.[7] are important, we are convinced that manometric studies of the muscles in the normal physiologic environment in vivo give clues to the underlying functional abnormalities (Table 9-1). The most convincing data have been presented by Bonavina et al.[6] and Migliore et al.[13]

In 1985 Bonavina et al.[6] showed that pharyngeal diverticula are only the tip of the iceberg and that a tailored surgical approach is effective. By means of esophageal manometry, pharyngeal pump failure, failure of cricopharyngeal relaxation-coordination, and cricopharyngeal hypertension were described as the main functional disorders associated with pharyngoesophageal dysphagia.

Migliore et al.[13] found that the resting tone of the upper esophageal sphincter in patients with Zenker's diverticulum was lower than normal, but the closing pressure and the duration of the postrelaxation contraction were higher. A similar finding was reported for the hypercontracting lower esophageal sphincter (LES).[14]

Table 9-1   Manometric abnormalities in patients with Zenker's diverticulum

Authors	Year	Abnormalities
Kodicek and Creamer[8]	1961	No abnormality found
Ellis et al.[9]	1969	Sphincteric coordination abnormalities
Hunt et al.[10]	1970	Elevated sphincter resting pressure
Pedersen et al.[11]	1973	No abnormality found
Knuff et al.[12]	1982	No abnormality found
Bonavina et al.[6]	1985	Pharyngeal pump failure, failure of cricopharyngeal relaxation, pharyngoesophageal incoordination, cricopharyngeal hypertension
Migliore et al.[13]	1994	Postrelaxation contraction, sphincteroesophageal incoordination

Migliore et al.[13] also detected pharyngoesophageal incoordination but stressed that sphincteroesophageal incoordination was an important phenomenon. Patients with diverticula therefore have stronger and longer-lasting upper esophageal peristaltic contractions.

In addition to functional esophageal studies, the further diagnostic workup includes x-ray studies for the exact location of the diverticulum. Endoscopy is needed to rule out an occasional rare cancer in diverticula (prevalence, 3%).[1]

A complete preoperative neurologic status of the cranial nerves is advisable to exclude laryngeal nerve palsy or other neurologic deficits (pharyngeal paralysis) that might lead to poor operative results.

Indication for Surgery

Surgery is needed to relieve the patient's symptoms of dysphagia, regurgitation, pain, coughing, weight loss, bad breath, and to eliminate the danger of aspiration and life-threatening pneumonia, especially in elderly patients. It is assumed that the larger the diverticulum, the more pronounced the symptoms of the patients should be.[7]

Surgical Approach

The historical development of interventions for Zenker's diverticulum began with external drainage (Bell in 1816, Nicoladoni in 1877, Wheeler in 1892, von Bergmann in 1892, and Kocher in 1892),[1] extended to invagination, then to excision, diverticulopexy, endoscopic diverticulostomy,[15,16] and finally cricopharyngeal myotomy.[1,17,18] Two-stage operations were in fashion in the second decade of this century (Goldmann in 1909, Murphy in 1916, and Judd in 1918).[1] These operations established a controlled fistula. The diverticulum was first closed, ligated, or attached to the skin before it was subsequently drained to the outside. At the time, these operations were able to reduce morbidity and mortality considerably. The modern era of antibiotic treatment initiated the comeback of one-stage operations (Sweet[17] in 1947 and Payne and Clagett[18] in 1960). Aubin[19] in 1936 was the first to suggest resection of a portion of the cricopharyngeal muscle, a technique that later became the standard method to treat the underlying functional disorder.[20]

Diverticulectomy

Simple excision of a hypopharyngeal diverticulum, originally the standard procedure, is still practiced in patients today.[17,18,21] However, it does not address the underlying functional problem. A longitudinal incision along the anterior border of the left sternocleidomastoid muscle is used to expose the pharynx and cervical esophagus. The sternocleidomastoid muscle and carotid sheath are retracted laterally and the trachea and larynx medially. Care is taken not to injure the recurrent laryngeal nerve. The diverticulum is dissected free from the surrounding tissue and the neck of the diverticulum is clearly demonstrated. Using a 60 F bougie or an endoscope, the original diameter of the esophagus is carefully preserved to avoid narrowing the esophagus and causing stenosis. The diverticular sac is removed with a conventional or endoscopic linear stapling device.[22] Laparoscopic instruments have the advantage of requiring less space and smaller incisions.[23] The cervical wound is closed without drainage and oral alimentation is begun the following day.

The mortality and morbidity of the procedure are considerable due, in part, to the old age and poor physiologic status of the patients. Mortality rates range from 0.4% to 8.3%[18,24] and morbidity rates vary from 6% to 53%.

Typical complications are recurrent nerve injury with difficulties in phonation, Horner's syndrome, hematoma, and septic complications such as abscess, wound infection, mediastinitis, and fistula. The recurrence rate of simple diverticulectomy depends on the length of follow-up and whether symptomatic and asymptomatic diverticula are included. The high recurrence rate of 16% reported in first postoperative year in a recent series[21] indicates that simple diverticulectomy alone does not solve the underlying functional problem.

Myotomy and Diverticulectomy or Diverticulopexy

A better understanding of pharyngoesophageal physiology and improved results after follow-up led to the use of cricopharyngeal myotomy.[6,25-28] Using a similar approach to diverticulectomy, the fibers of the cricopharyngeal muscle, located inferior to the neck of the diverticulum, are divided down to the mucosa. The myotomy is extended cephalad to the diverticular neck by dividing 1 to 2 cm of the inferior constrictor muscle of the pharynx and caudally by dividing the muscle fibers of the cervical esophagus for a length of 4 to 5 cm. When complete, the mucosa bulges freely through the myotomized muscle without being restricted by small bands. As a consequence of the myotomy, most small diverticula disappear so that myotomy alone will suffice. Those diverticula that do not disappear can be excised or suspended to the prevertebral fascia or to the pharynx as cranially as possible. This largely avoids the typical septic complications that develop when the mucosa is breached. Therefore, if anatomically possible, diverticulopexy rather than diverticulectomy is the preferred approach. Up to 85% excellent results can be expected using this technique, especially when manometric abnormalities have been demonstrated.[6] The recurrence rate in large series is approximately 5%.[27]

Endoscopic Sphincterotomy

The endoscopic approach to diverticula has been resurrected by the recent availability of linear stapling devices for laparoscopic surgery.[2,16,17,22] Originally described by Mosher[15] in 1917, the endoscopic procedure of esophagodiverticulostomy (dividing the common wall between the diverticulum and the esophageal lumen) was applied successfully in 100 patients by Dohlmann and Mattsson.[16] Despite the elegance of the procedure because of its brevity and simplicity, the inherent problems are the risk of mediastinal infection and the need for multiple procedures to relieve symptoms in a considerable number of patients.[24] Broader application of endoscopic stapling devices with better prevention of cervical or mediastinal infection may improve the results of endoscopic esophagodiverticulostomy.

In summary, several surgical options for the treatment for Zenker's diverticulum are available. We use open cricomyotomy and diverticulopexy as the procedure of choice. A randomized trial comparing this approach to endoscopic technique is now timely. The relevant end points for such a trial would be safety, feasibility, benefit, and level of discomfort for the patient.

ESOPHAGEAL BODY DIVERTICULA

The underlying functional disorder in midesophageal or epiphrenic diverticula still must be fully elucidated. The term "esophageal folklore" has been used to describe functional studies.[29] Preoperative physiologic studies are, however, essential because resection of a diverticulum without prior knowledge of the pathophysiology and without performing a concomitant long myotomy almost invariably leads to recurrence. Midesophageal or epiphrenic diverticula occur less frequently than hypopharyngeal diverticula with a ratio of 1 to 5.[30] The lower prevalence is, in part, due to the fact that only a minority of them (20% to 25%) are symptomatic or are even detected.[31]

Anatomy and Physiology

Originally Mondière[32] suggested that pulsion diverticula were mucosal herniations through the muscular wall and caused a certain degree of obstruction leading to characteristic symptoms.[31] The introduction and improvement of manometry techniques revealed that some form of motility disorder is at least in part a causal factor. This motor abnormality produces a functional distal obstruction together with an intraluminal pressure rise. The latter are recorded manometrically as pathologic contractions of varying morphology. Achalasia, diffuse esophageal spasm, or related motor disorders, such as nutcracker esophagus, or severe nonspecific motility disorders may be the underlying cause or common denominator of this condition. Surprisingly, only a minority of these patients develop diverticula.[33,34]

It has become the principle of modern functional surgery to identify the underlying disorder and to tailor the surgical intervention to treat the disease in an optimal and effective manner.[35,36]

Symptoms

The spectrum of symptoms of esophageal diverticula is very broad.[30,37] In the majority of patients, the diverticulum is an incidental finding on a barium swallow examination or upper gastrointestinal endoscopy. These patients often report no symptoms or have mild dysphagia. Other patients may complain of incapacitating symptoms, such as severe dysphagia, chest pain, food retention, bad breath, regurgitation, and aspiration, which can lead to life-threatening pneumonia. The degree of neuromuscular dysfunction and the size of the diverticulum do not seem to correlate well with symptoms.

Functional and Imaging Diagnostic Studies

DeMeester[35] demonstrated that better functional esophageal studies, such as stationary and ambulatory esophageal manometry and pH-monitoring of the foregut, lead to better results of surgery. Barium swallow is usually the initial step to diagnose suspected esophageal diverticulum and segmental spasm with compartmentalization of the esophagus. It may provide some clues as to the associated motility disorder and will exclude other lesions such as cancer or stricture. Endoscopy is the next step to evaluate the condition because it allows more detailed inspection of the size, location, and mucosal status of the diverticulum. Preoperative manometry is the key diagnostic test to identify motor disorders of the esophageal body or lower sphincter. Diffuse esophageal spasm, vigorous achalasia, and nonspecific motor disorders are commonly associated with diverticula.

In most patients with a diverticulum, an abnormality of the esophageal body or lower sphincter can be identified manometrically[23] (Table 9-2). The recent in-

Table 9-2 Manometric abnormalities in patients with esophageal body diverticula

Authors	Year	Abnormalities
Evander et al.[34]	1986	Simultaneous, tertiary, repetitive contractions and aperistalsis
Mulder et al.[31]	1989	Achalasia-like pattern
Eypasch et al.[38]	1992	Simultaneous and repetitive contractions
Streitz et al.[39]	1992	Simultaneous and prolonged contractions
Altorki et al.[37]	1993	Patterns like achalasia, diffuse spasm, and hypertensive lower sphincter

troduction of 24-hour ambulatory esophageal manometry has greatly simplified the identification of motility disorders in patients with chest pain and dysphagia.[40] The motility abnormality may be intermittent and can therefore be missed by stationary manometry but is detected with the continuous ambulatory recording technique. Twenty-four–hour esophageal pH monitoring is essential to rule out pathologic gastroesophageal reflux.

Treatment

The principle of modern functional esophageal surgery is to identify the underlying motility disorder and to tailor the surgical intervention accordingly.[35] Surgical interventions have a clear-cut indication and are based on physiologic data about the underlying motor disorder.[38] The decision to operate depends on the balance of the patient's symptoms, diet, lifestyle adjustments, and nutritional status.

"Masterful inactivity" in asymptomatic or mildly disturbing diverticula is a good practice.[29] Large pouches with the threat of aspiration, especially in the elderly and less compliant patients, require surgical treatment.[37] In the era of thoracoendoscopic techniques, surgery for a benign condition that usually does not threaten the patient's life must not become a playground for hyperactive surgeons.[41] Endoscopic staplers and devices must not become a temptation to widen the indication for surgery because this inevitably results in a bad outcome for some patients.

Surgical Approach

The preoperative preparation of the patient includes careful emptying of large diverticula by nasogastric aspiration to avoid aspiration during the induction of anesthesia.

We recommend the following standardized transthoracic approach.[38] Preoperative imaging studies are mandatory to locate the side of the diverticulum exactly because this dictates the side of thoracotomy. Usually a left thoracotomy in the sixth intercostal space is performed. After incision of the mediastinal pleura, the esophagus is located and the diverticulum is dissected free of surrounding tissue. Care is taken not to injure the mucosa. A nasogastric tube, a bougie, or an endoscope can help to identify the esophagus. Perforation of the esophagus or the diverticulum should be avoided. Once the diverticulum is located and isolated, we prefer to excise it by dividing the neck with a stapling device. A clamp applied on the diverticulum should avoid spillage of contents into the chest. Smaller midesophageal diverticula may be inverted or suspended to the prevertebral fascia. After resection of the pouch, the muscular wall defect is carefully closed using fine sutures. The mobilized esophagus is rotated and a long myotomy is performed on the opposite side of the diverticulum, extending from the aortic arch down to the stomach. Physiologic data indicate that distal functional obstruction that leads to a rise in intraluminal pressure is a major cause of recurrent mucosal herniation. To relieve obstruction and reduce outflow resistance, the myotomy should extend across the lower esophageal sphincter onto the stomach.[38] A 2 cm incision is made in the phrenoesophageal membrane along the left diaphragmatic crus and a flap of gastric fundus is pulled into the chest. The fat pad on the exposed gastroesophageal junction is removed and the myotomy is extended distally for 1 to 2 cm below the junction. The cardia is reconstructed by suturing the tongue of gastric fundus to the margins of the myotomy for a distance of 4 cm in an attempt to provide adequate antireflux control. Different approaches spare the lower sphincter if it functions normally on manometric evaluation.[39]

RESULTS OF SURGICAL TREATMENT

An overview of recent series of patients with esophageal diverticula associated with motor abnormalities underscores the fact that both the disease and the need

Table 9-3   Esophageal diverticula: Results of surgical treatment

Authors	Year	No. of Patients	Diagnosis Technique	Grading of Results
Evander et al.[34]	1986	9	Various EMD Diverticulectomy Diverticulopexy Myotomy, AR	7/9 Good 2/9 Occasional sticking
Mulder et al.[31]	1989	4	Achalasia Diverticulectomy 1/4 Nissen	3/4 Good 1/4 Fair
Streitz et al.[39]	1992	16	Various EMD Diverticulectomy Tailored myotomy	14/16 Excellent 2/16 Good
Eypasch et al.[38]	1992	19	Diffuse esophageal spasm Myotomy, diverticulectomy Esophagectomy	8/14 Excellent 5/14 Good 1/14 No change
D'Ugo et al.[42]	1992	19	Various EMD Myotomy	Satisfactory relief
Peracchia et al.[41]	1992	5	Various EMD Diverticulectomy	4/5 Excellent 1/5 Reoperation
Benacci et al.[30]	1993	33	Various EMD Diverticulectomy Diverticulopexy Myotomy	14/29 Excellent 8/29 Good 5/29 Fair 2/29 Poor
Altorki et al.[37]	1993	17	Various EMD Diverticulectomy Diverticulopexy Myotomy, Belsey	13/14 Excellent 1/14 Poor
Hudspeth et al.[43]	1993	9	Various EMD Diverticulectomy Myotomy	9/9 Good/Excellent

EMD = esophageal motor disorder; AR = antireflux procedure.

for surgical intervention are uncommon* (Table 9-3). Most of the recent series report excellent to good results in 75% to 95% of patients. However, one fourth to one third of patients are not completely satisfied with the results of the operation, which indicates a need for further diagnostic and therapeutic refinements. It should be emphasized that the system of reporting operative results as "excellent, good, fair, and poor" is very crude and subjective. In some series, a very unfavorable outcome was reported after conservative treatment of diverticula. This prompted the authors to advise surgical intervention for diverticula to avoid aspiration and pneumonia and life-threatening situations.[37] Orringer,[29] however, recommends the "masterful inactivity" approach with respect to mildly symptomatic or asymptomatic esophageal diverticula.

CONCLUSION

Unsatisfactory results indicate incomplete understanding of physiology and an inadequate surgical approach to the disease. Ambulatory recording techniques have recently become available and have refined the classification of esophageal motor dysfunction.[39,44] Esophageal diverticula may be just a facet of a more complex motility disorder involving the entire foregut, and further knowledge will help to tailor the surgical treatment to the individual patient. Endoscopic surgery and its technical innovations such as staplers have opened the door to the treatment of esophageal diverticula and motor disorders by minimally invasive techniques. The temptation to treat patients endoscopically and in a presumably elegant way should not undermine the strict indication for surgery. Just because surgeons have a new hammer, every esophageal problem must not become a nail.

---

*References 30, 31, 34, 37-39, and 41-43.

REFERENCES

1. Grégoire J, Duranceau A. Surgical management of Zenker's diverticulum. Hepatogastroenterology 39:32-138, 1992.
2. Broll R, Kramer T, Kalb K, Bruch HP. Das Zenker'sche Divertikel—Langzeitergebnisse nach operativer Therapie. Chirurg 62:668-672, 1991.
3. Overbeek JJM. Meditation on the pathogenesis of hypopharyngeal (Zenker's) diverticulum and a report of endoscopic treatment in 545 patients. Ann Otol Rhinol Laryngol 103:178-185, 1994.
4. Zenker FA, von Ziemssen H. Krankheiten des Oesophagus. In von Ziemssen H, ed. Handbuch der speziellen Pathologie und Therapie, 7. Leipzig: C Vogel, 1877, 30 q.
5. Rosetti M, Siewert R. Oesophagusdivertikel. In Siewert R, Blum AL, Waldeck F, eds. Funktionsstörungen der Speiseröhre. Berlin, Heidelberg, New York: Springer, 1976, p 183.
6. Bonavina L, Khan NA, DeMeester TR. Pharyngoesophageal dysfunctions. Arch Surg 120:541-549, 1985.
7. Lerut T, van Raemdonck D, Guelinckx P, Dom R, Geboes K. Zenker's diverticulum: Is myotomy of the cricopharyngeus useful? How long should it be? Hepatogastroenterology 39:127-131, 1992.
8. Kodicek J, Creamer B. A study of pharyngeal pouches. J Laryngol Otol 75:406-411, 1961.
9. Ellis FH, Schlegel JF, Lynch VP, Payne WS. Cricopharyngeal myotomy for pharyngo-esophageal diverticulum. Ann Surg 170:340-349, 1969.

10. Hunt PS, Connel AM, Smiley TB. The cricopharyngeal sphincter in gastric reflux. Gut 11:303-306, 1970.
11. Pedersen SA, Hansen JB, Alstrup P. Pharyngo-esophageal diverticula. Scand J Thorac Cardiovasc Surg 7:87-90, 1973.
12. Knuff TE, Benjamin SB, Castell DO. Pharyngoesophageal (Zenker's) diverticulum: A reappraisal. Gastroenterology 82:734-736, 1982.
13. Migliore M, Payne H, Jeyasingham K. Pathophysiologic basis for operation on Zenker's diverticulum. Ann Thorac Surg 57:1616-1621, 1994.
14. Eypasch E, DeMeester TR, Stein H, Vestweber KH, Barlow AP, Jenkins H. Hypercontracting lower esophageal sphincter as a cause of dysphagia and chest pain. In Skinner DB, Little AG, Ferguson MK, eds. Diseases of the Esophagus. New York: Futura Publishing Co., 1989, pp 343-353.
15. Mosher HP. Webs and pouches of the esophagus, their diagnosis and treatment. Surg Gynecol Obstet 25:175-187, 1917.
16. Dohlmann G, Mattsson O. Endoscopic treatment of the hypopharyngeal diverticula. Arch Otolaryngol 71:744-752, 1960.
17. Sweet RH. Excision of diverticulum of pharyngo-esophageal junction and lower esophagus by means of one-stage procedure. Ann Surg 143:433-438, 1956.
18. Payne WS, Clagett OT. Pharyngeal and esophageal diverticula. Curr Probl Surg 2:1-31, 1965.
19. Aubin A. Un cas de diverticule de pulsion de l'oesophage traité par la résection de la poche associée à l'oesophagotomie extramuqueuse. Ann Otolaryngol 2:167-177, 1936.
20. Belsey R. Functional diseases of the esophagus. J Thorac Cardiovasc Surg 52:164-188, 1966.
21. Aggerholm K, Illum P. Surgical treatment of Zenker's diverticulum. J Laryngol Otol 104:312-314, 1990.
22. Collard JM, Otte JB, Kestens PJ. Endoscopic stapling technique of esophagodiverticulostomy for Zenker's diverticulum. Ann Thorac Surg 56:573-576, 1993.
23. Spiro SA, Berg HM. Applying the endoscopic stapler in excision of Zenker's diverticulum: A solution for two intraoperative problems. Otolaryngol Head Neck Surg 110:603-604, 1994.
24. Bowdler DA, Stell PM. Surgical management of posterior pharyngeal pulsion diverticula: Inversion versus one-stage excision. Br J Surg 74:988-990, 1987.
25. Laccourreye O, Ménard M, Cauchois R, Huart J, Jouffre V, Brasnu D, Laccourreye H. Esophageal diverticulum: Diverticulopexy versus diverticulectomy. Laryngoscope 104:889-892, 1994.
26. Payne WS. The treatment of pharyngoesophageal diverticulum: The simple and the complex. Hepatogastroenterology 39:109-114, 1992.
27. Moran ADG, Wilson AJ, Muhanna AH. Pharyngeal diverticula. Clin Otolaryngol 11:219-225, 1986.
28. Wayman DM, Byl FM, Adour KK. Endoscopic diverticulotomy for the treatment of Zenker's diverticulum. Otolaryngol Head Neck Surg 104:448-452, 1991.
29. Orringer MB. Epiphrenic diverticula: Fact and fable. Ann Thorac Surg 55:1067-1068, 1993.
30. Benacci JC, Deschamps C, Trastek VF, Allen MS, Daly RC, Pairolero PC. Epiphrenic diverticulum: Results of surgical treatment. Ann Thorac Surg 55:1109-1114, 1993.
31. Mulder DG, Rosenkranz E, DenBesten L. Management of huge esophageal diverticula. Am J Surg 157:303-307, 1989.
32. Mondière JT. Notes sur quelques maladies de l'oesophage. Arch Gen Med Paris 3:28-65, 1833.
33. Fekete F, Vonns C. Surgical management of esophageal thoracic diverticula. Hepatogastroenterology 39:97-99, 1992.
34. Evander A, Little AG, Ferguson MK, Skinner DB. Diverticula of the mid- and lower esophagus: Pathogenesis and surgical management. World J Surg 10:820-828, 1986.
35. DeMeester TR. Surgery for esophageal motor disorders. Ann Thorac Surg 34:225-229, 1982.
36. Attwood SEA, Eypasch EP, DeMeester TR. Surgical therapies for dysphagia. In Gelfand DW, Richter JE, eds. Diagnosis and Treatment of Dysphagia. New York: Igaku-Shoin Publishing Co., 1989, pp 335-370.
37. Altorki NK, Sunagawa M, Skinner DB. Thoracic esophageal diverticula—Why is operation necessary. J Thorac Cardiovasc Surg 105:260-264, 1993.

38. Eypasch EP, DeMeester TR, Klingman RR, Stein HJ. Physiologic assessment and surgical management of diffuse esophageal spasm. J Thorac Cardiovasc Surg 104:859-869, 1992.
39. Streitz JM, Glick ME, Ellis FH. Selective use of myotomy for treatment of epiphrenic diverticula. Arch Surg 127:585-588, 1992.
40. Eypasch E, Stein HJ, DeMeester TR, Johansson KE, Barlow AP, Schneider GT. Ambulatory 24-hour esophageal motility monitoring: A new technique to define and clarify esophageal motor disorders. Am J Surg 159:144-151, 1990.
41. Peracchia A, Ancona E, Ruol A, Bardini R, Segalin A, Bonavina L. Use of mini-invasive procedures in esophageal surgery. Chirurgie 118:305-309, 1992.
42. D'Ugo D, Cardillo G, Granone P, Coppola R, Margaritora S, Picciocchi A. Esophageal diverticula. Physiological basis for surgical management. J Cardiothorac Surg 6:330-334, 1992.
43. Hudspeth DA, Thorne MT, Conroy R, Pennell TC. Management of epiphrenic esophageal diverticula—A fifteen year experience. Am Surg 59:40-42, 1993.
44. Stein H, DeMeester TR, Eypasch E, Klingman RR. Ambulatory 24-hour esophageal manometry in the evaluation of esophageal motor disorders and non-cardiac chest pain. Surgery 110:753-763, 1991.

10

Cricopharyngeal Myotomy for Neurologic Dysphagia

Nancy Claire Poirier, M.D. • *Raymond Taillefer,* M.D.
André Duranceau, M.D.

The voluntary oral phase of deglutition is controlled by the cerebral cortex and the brain stem. The involuntary pharyngeal phase is regulated by the brain stem. Dysfunction of the central nervous system or interruption of either sensory or motor transport pathways at the peripheral level can result in oropharyngeal dysphagia. The clinical presentation may vary and is influenced by the location of the damage and its extent. Hesitation and inability to initiate swallowing or inability to move food or liquid from the mouth to the pharyngeal cavity reflects dysfunction of the tongue, soft palate, or suprahyoid muscles. Poor transport from the pharynx to esophagus suggests dysfunction at the pharyngoesophageal junction. When oropharyngeal dysphagia occurs in response to voluntary deglutitions, misdirection of the food bolus usually causes symptoms by its misorientation: pharyngo-oral regurgitation, pharyngonasal regurgitation, laryngeal penetration, or tracheo-bronchial aspiration.

Cricopharyngeal myotomy is the only operation that is documented to decrease the difficulties in transport from pharynx to esophagus in this difficult category of oropharyngeal dysphagia patients.

This chapter examines subjective and objective responses of patients with neurologic dysphagia treated by cricopharyngeal myotomy. In addition, the existing surgical literature is reviewed and prognostic factors for improvement are identified.

MATERIAL AND METHODS

Twenty patients (10 women and 10 men) were evaluated for oropharyngeal dysphagia resulting from neurologic disease. Symptoms were present for an average period of 25 months (range, 2 to 84 months). Fifteen patients had sequelae of cerebrovascular accidents. The remainder of the patient population included one patient with cerebral and upper cervical spine trauma, one patient with amyotrophic lateral sclerosis, and one patient with Parkinson's disease. One patient had postoperative dysphagia following posterior fossa surgery for an acoustic neuroma. A final patient had oropharyngeal symptoms from a pseudobulbar palsy. Ages ranged from 35 to 82 years (average, 68 years). Upper esophageal function was assessed before and after cricopharyngeal myotomy. Follow-up ranged from 1 to 120 months (mean, 35 months).

Operation

All patients underwent cricopharyngeal myotomy using a standardized technique.[1] A left cervical oblique incision was used along the anteromedial border of the sternomastoid muscle (Fig. 10-1). A 36 F mercury bougie was passed into the

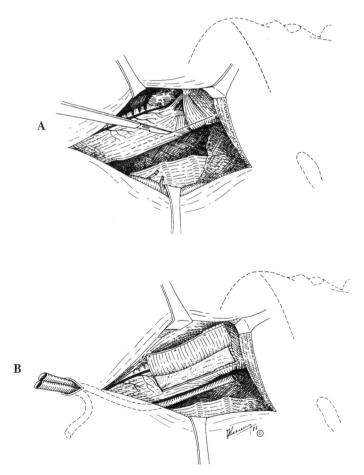

Fig. 10-1 A, The pharyngoesophageal junction is everted toward the left. The myotomy is begun on the right and dissection is carried between mucosa and muscularis. **B,** A 6 cm myotomy is completed with proximal and distal transverse transsection, creating a flap of muscle that is resected for histologic evaluation.

esophagus and used as a stent. A 6 cm myotomy was performed on the postero-lateral aspect of the pharyngoesophageal junction. The muscularis along the myotomy was dissected free from the submucosa. A flap of muscle was created by proximal and distal transverse transection and resected for histologic analysis. A nasogastric tube was left in place for gastric decompression until peristalsis was observed. Penrose drains were used in the thoracic inlet and behind the myotomized zone. They were left in place for 24 hours. A liquid diet was begun on the first postoperative day. Patients were usually discharged on the second or third postoperative day.

Radiology

Barium esophagrams were obtained under fluoroscopic observation. Radiographs were obtained with four to six frames printed per second. Identification of voluntary deglutition, swallowing hesitation, pharyngeal stasis, functional obstruction and incoordination at the upper esophageal sphincter (UES) level, epiglottic dysfunction, and tracheal aspirations were recorded.

Manometry

Manometric assessment of the pharyngoesophageal junction was obtained in 16 patients using a perfused system. Both standard recording catheters (10 patients) and the Dent sleeve probe for the UES (five patients) were used for recording of the pharyngoesophageal junction before and after the operation. Our standard recording catheter (Mui Scientific, Toronto, Ontario) is a four-lumen catheter where each lumen ends in a lateral port. Each port is oriented at 90 degrees and at 5 cm from each other. During recording one port is located in the pharynx, one in the high pressure zone between the pharynx and the esophagus, and the last two are in the cervical esophagus. The 6 cm Dent sleeve probe is similarly positioned at the pharyngoesophageal junction so two ports are in the hypopharynx 2 cm apart from each other and a distal perfusion channel is in the cervical esophagus. Both systems are perfused by a pneumohydraulic pump generating a pressure of 15 psi. Relaxation of the UES is considered complete when the UES resting pressure drops to within 5 mm Hg of the cervical esophageal baseline. The UES is interpreted as being coordinated when the UES relaxation period completely encompasses the pharyngeal contraction duration and when the peak pharyngeal contraction concurs with the nadir of UES relaxation. Mean values recorded during 10 voluntary deglutitions were calculated. These values and their standard deviations were compared before and after the operation.

Radionuclide Hypopharyngeal Emptying Study

Pharyngeal emptying scintiscans were obtained in six patients both pre- and postoperatively. A single bolus of 0.1 mCi technetium 99m diluted in 10 ml of water was used. The percentage of radioactivity retained in the hypopharynx was calculated at 2, 5, 15, 30, 45, 60, 90, and 120 seconds. The presence of pharyngonasal and pharyngo-oral regurgitation and tracheobronchial aspiration was computed.

Statistical Analysis

A two-tailed Student's t test for paired values and chi-squared analysis for discontinuous values were used when appropriate. A p value of less than 0.05 was considered significant.

RESULTS
Clinical Presentation

The clinical findings are summarized in Table 10-1. All 20 patients initially presented with dysphagia at the oropharyngeal level. Three of the 20 patients were completely relieved of this dysphagia after the operation and 11 patients were improved. Dysphagia was considered unchanged in six patients. Pharyngo-oral and/or pharyngonasal regurgitation was observed preoperatively in eight and seven patients, respectively, and seven patients experienced either complete or partial relief after surgery. Eighteen of the 20 patients presented with aspiration episodes. After cricopharyngeal myotomy, 11 patients presented no clinical evidence of aspiration, while four other patients reported fewer aspiration episodes. Three patients were not relieved of their aspiration symptoms after surgery. Two of these patients subsequently underwent laryngeal exclusion, and a gastrostomy was performed in the third patient. There were no postoperative complications and no mortality resulted from the operation.

Radiology

The radiologic observations are detailed in Table 10-2. Inability to swallow (apraxia) and delayed bolus propulsion persisted postoperatively in two patients. In two other patients, oral phase dysfunction became more evident in the postoperative evaluation. Epiglottic dysfunction was initially observed in five patients and it was seen in six patients postoperatively. Functional obstruction at the UES level was documented in 16 patients. After the operation, 13 of these 16 patients showed improved radiologic transit. Only three of 11 patients with pharyngeal stasis on preoperative esophagrams showed complete emptying after cricopharyngeal myotomy. Stasis was recorded in two patients only after the myotomy. Aspiration was present in nine patients preoperatively and eight patients postoperatively.

Manometry

Table 10-3 details pre- and postoperative manometric results using standard manometric recordings and the Dent sleeve technique. The pharyngeal resting pressures, contraction pressures, and contraction duration remained unchanged after the myotomy. The UES resting pressures and the duration of relaxation were

Table 10-1   Clinical presentation in 20 patients

Symptoms	Preoperative (n = 20)	Postoperative (n = 20)	p Value
Dysphagia	20	17	NS
Aspiration	18	7	0.03
Regurgitations			
Pharyngo-oral	8	4	NS
Pharyngonasal	7	4	NS
Voluntary deglutition	19	18	NS
Dysarthria	4	4	NS

NS = not significant.

Table 10-2   Radiologic findings

Observations	Preoperative (n = 20)	Postoperative (n = 20)	p Value
Swallowing apraxia	3	4	NS
Pharyngeal stasis	11	10	NS
Functional obstruction of UES	16	3	0.001
Epiglottic incoordination	5	6	NS
Aspirations	9	8	NS

NS = not significant.

Table 10-3   Manometric data

Parameters	Preoperative (n = 10)	Postoperative (n = 10)	p Value
Single port			
Pharyngeal			
Resting pressure (mm Hg)	3.8 ± 3.9	5.3 ± 5.9	NS
Contraction pressure (mm Hg)	21.4 ± 11.0	18.9 ± 11.6	NS
Contraction time (sec)	0.8 ± 0.2	0.9 ± 0.3	NS
Upper esophageal sphincter			
Resting pressure (mm Hg)	52.4 ± 35.0	22.8 ± 17.0	0.01
Contraction pressure (mm Hg)	73.9 ± 40.4	40.3 ± 31.3	NS
Relaxation time (sec)	1.8 ± 1.0	1.2 ± 0.4	0.04
Coordination	0.2 ± 0.3	0.1 ± 0.2	NS
Dent sleeve			
Upper esophageal sphincter			
Resting pressure (mm Hg)	56.6 ± 28.2	34.4 ± 18.8	—

NS = not significant.

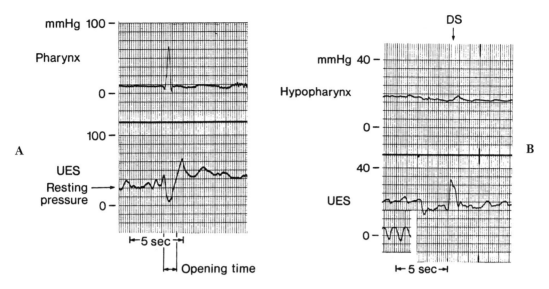

Fig. 10-2 A, Normal contraction of the pharynx with normal relaxation of the UES. **B,** Very weak pharyngeal contraction with absent relaxation of the UES in a patient who had a cerebrovascular accident.

Table 10-4 Hypopharyngeal radionuclide transit study

Observations	Preoperative (n = 6)	Postoperative (n = 6)
Retention at 120 seconds	6	6
% Retention	16 ± 12	14 ± 9
Regurgitation	6	4
Pharyngo-oral	4	4
Pharyngonasal	1	2
Aspiration	4	1

both significantly decreased by the operation. The Dent sleeve pressure readings in five patients showed a decrease in UES resting pressures but no statistical analysis was attempted because of the limited number of observations. Manometric recording values showed the same variation whether the recordings were made using a single-port system or the Dent sleeve technique. UES incoordination is a constant observation and remained unchanged after the operation (Fig. 10-2).

Radionuclide Hypopharyngeal Emptying Study

Six patients had pre- and postoperative emptying scintiscans with liquids (Table 10-4). The hypopharyngeal retention of radioactive material over a 2-minute period is plotted in Fig. 10-3. Hypopharyngeal stasis persisted after surgery. Episodes of pharyngo-oral and pharyngonasal regurgitation were unchanged. Tracheal

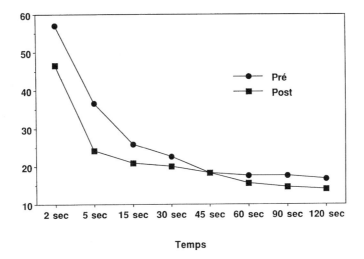

Fig. 10-3 Liquid-emptying scintiscan at the pharyngoesophageal junction. Hypopharyngeal stasis is unchanged after myotomy when using a single-liquid bolus.

aspiration seen in four patients before cricopharyngeal myotomy was documented in one patient after the operation.

DISCUSSION

More than 242 cricopharyngeal myotomies have been reported for the treatment of neurogenic oropharyngeal dysphagia in the English literature. Most of these studies are case reports and contain little objective data, which makes it difficult to draw conclusions as to the true efficacy of this procedure. In a recent review of 201 cases, 50% of the patients who were operated on were reported to have satisfactory to excellent results.[2]

Stroke is probably the most common neurologic cause of dysphagia. Damage resulting from a cerebrovascular accident can be varied, provoking a number of swallowing disorders. Severe persistent dysphagia from lesions localized in one hemisphere is rare.[3,4] Manifestations can be limited to the oral phase with poor lingual control. This inadequate tongue propulsion can affect the early pharyngeal phase by delaying reflex initiation of a swallow and reducing pharyngeal peristalsis.[5] Localized lesions of the brain stem can be manifested by isolated pharyngeal paralysis and UES achalasia.[6] Functional recovery is especially good in these patients. One study recorded normal swallowing in 86% of patients 2 weeks after an acute unilateral stroke.[4]

In the surgical literature, 54 patients with persistent oropharyngeal dysphagia resulting from brain damage caused by vascular lesions were treated by cricopharyngeal myotomy.[7-25] Damage varied considerably and there was lack of uniformity in the response to surgical treatment. Lacunar lesions of the brain stem and basilar artery thrombosis were associated with good functional results. Overall, 13 of 54 patients showed excellent results, while 22 were improved. The remainder of the group were found to have unchanged symptoms over time. The postoperative mortality was 12% and was mainly a consequence of cardiopulmonary complications. Morbidity resulted mostly from continued aspiration.

Of our 20 patients, 80% had cerebral damage from vascular lesions. In this subset of patients, the myotomy seems to alleviate a degree of functional obstruction caused by the uncoordinated UES. Although radiologic, manometric, and radionuclide evaluations show persistence of dysfunction with pharyngeal stasis, the myotomy seems to allow an easier transit of the food bolus toward the cervical esophagus. The significant decrease in UES resting pressures and the decrease in opening time of the sphincter during pharyngeal contraction suggest that the myotomy results in a decreased resistance to pharyngoesophageal transit.

Five of our 20 patients experienced no change in their symptoms after surgery. This subgroup of patients included one patient with each of the following conditions: amyotrophic lateral sclerosis, Parkinson's disease, and cerebral and cervical spine trauma. The two other patients had strokes. One had a lacunar bulbar cerebrovascular accident and one had a left hemispheric cerebrovascular accident. All five patients presented with dysarthria and/or absent voluntary deglutition. Our experience in this regard is supported by others who report that when oral phase dysfunction predominates, the response to cricopharyngeal myotomy is uncertain.[6,13]

In amyotrophic lateral sclerosis, degeneration of motoneurons in the brain, brain stem, and spinal cord occurs. Dysphagia results when nerves are damaged, exhibiting deglutition dysfunction mainly of the oral phase and during the early pharyngeal phase. Muscles of the tongue and hypopharynx show progressive signs of denervation with manifestations ranging from paresis, atrophy, and fasciculations to complete loss of voluntary deglutition. It has been suggested that the inappropriate tongue movement delays the triggering of the swallowing reflex.[26] Thus the pharyngeal phase is incoordinated and the UES is not relaxed. As a result, eating time is long and laborious. Food and secretions accumulate in the mouth and aspiration invariably occurs. Cricopharyngeal myotomy for amyotrophic lateral sclerosis does not consistently help these patients since the oral phase dysfunction predominates and is not modified by this surgical intervention. Loizou, Small, and Dalton[27] reported an initial improvement in 19 of 25 patients but their operative mortality was 20%. Lebo, Kwei Sang, and Norris[28,29] reported that 6 months after operation, 50% of their patients still showed progressive amelioration in their swallowing.

Parkinson's disease can also result in deglutition abnormalities characterized by oral phase dysfunction. Lingual hesitancy and poor control of bolus propulsion toward the pharynx may cause symptoms similar to those of patients with amyotrophic lateral sclerosis.[30] A good clinical response was obtained in six of seven patients who underwent cricopharyngeal myotomy.[10,19,31]

Conflicting results are seen in patients with oropharyngeal dysphagia resulting from trauma and peripheral nerve lesions. Henderson et al.[32] and Mills[13] reported excellent results following myotomy, whereas Akl and Blakeley[31] observed little improvement. Dysphagia from brain stem compression caused by a tumor or aneurysm was reported to be improved with the ablation of the lesion.[13,32]

Response of dysphagia caused by bulbar poliomyelitis, progressive bulbar palsy, and pseudopalsy treated by cricopharyngeal myotomy has been reported in 14 patients.* These patients manifested mainly pharyngeal phase disorders. Two showed excellent results after myotomy, including one patient from our group. Seven patients were improved and symptoms were unchanged in two patients.

CONCLUSION

What are the most reliable criteria for a successful cricopharyngeal myotomy in patients with neurogenic dysphagia? Many patients, specifically stroke victims, regain oral feedings without aspiration spontaneously or through feeding reeducation. Any surgical intervention, including cricopharyngeal myotomy, therefore should be delayed for at least 6 months after the neurologic event. Cricopharyngeal myotomy can be undertaken with reasonable expectation for success if the following conditions coexist: (1) normal voluntary deglutition; (2) adequate tongue movement; (3) intact laryngeal function and phonation; and (4) absence of dysarthria. These observations are supported by Bergman and Lewicki[6] and Mills,[13] who reported that intact voluntary deglutition seems essential, while poor propulsion by the posterior tongue and hypopharynx reduces the value of myotomy. Moreover, Wiles[38] affirms that cricopharyngeal myotomy is pointless if the cause is essentially at the oral or early pharyngeal phase. For these reasons, laryngeal diversion or complete laryngectomy with permanent tracheostomy can be the intervention of choice in patients with severe laryngeal dysfunction and in whom no improvement is anticipated.[16] The criteria for selection are based on strict assessment of symptoms, radiologic and radionuclide transit observations, and manometric evaluation.

---

*References 14, 17, 18, 20, 21, 27, and 33-37.

REFERENCES

1. Duranceau AC, Jamieson GG, Beauchamp G. The techniques of cricopharyngeal myotomy. Surg Clin North Am 63:833-839, 1983.
2. Duranceau A. Pharyngeal and cricopharyngeal disorders. In Pearson FG, ed. Esophageal Surgery. New York: Churchill Livingstone, 1995, pp 389-415.
3. Meadows JC. Dysphagia in unilateral cerebral lesions. J Neurol Neurosurg Psychiatry 36:853-860, 1973.
4. Gordon C, Langton Hewer R, Wade DT. Dysphagia in acute stroke. Br Med J 295:411-414, 1987.
5. Veis S, Logemann J. The nature of swallowing disorders in CVA patients. Arch Phys Med Rehabil 66:372-375, 1985.
6. Bergman AB, Lewicki AM. Complete esophageal obstruction from cricopharyngeal achalasia. Radiology 123:289-290, 1977.
7. Ellis FH, Crozier RE. Cervical esophageal dysphagia in indications for and results of cricopharyngeal myotomy. Ann Surg 194:279-289, 1981.
8. Gagic NM. Cricopharyngeal myotomy. Can J Surg 26:47-49, 1983.
9. Desaulty A, Piquet JJ, Vaneecloo FM, Decroix G. Interêt de la myotomie du cricopharyngien et des fibres supérieures de l'oesophage dans les dyskinesies pharyngo-oesophagiennes. J Fr Otorhinolaryngol 24:527-535, 1975.

10. West EM, Baker HW. Esophageal dysphagia treated by cricopharyngeal myotomy. Am Surg 43:703-708, 1977.
11. Hirano M. Cricopharyngeal myotomy for paralytic dysphagia. J FRORL 23:731-734, 1974.
12. Blakeley WR, Gerety EJ, Smith DE. Section of the cricopharyngeus muscle for dysphagia. Arch Surg 96:745-762, 1968.
13. Mills CP. Dysphagia in pharyngeal paralysis treated by cricopharyngeal sphincterotomy. Lancet 1:455-457, 1973.
14. Lund WS. The cricopharyngeal sphincter: Its relationship to the relief of pharyngeal paralysis and the surgical treatment of the early pharyngeal pouch. J Laryngol Otol 82:353-367, 1968.
15. Wilkins SA. Indications for section of the cricopharyngeus muscle. Am J Surg 108:533-538, 1964.
16. Butcher RB. Treatment of chronic aspirations as a complication of cerebrovascular accident. Laryngoscope 92:681-685, 1982.
17. Van Overbeek JJM, Betlem HC. Cricopharyngeal myotomy in pharyngeal paralysis: Cineradiographic and manometric indications. Ann Otol 88:596-602, 1979.
18. Calcaterra TC, Kadell BM, Ward PH. Dysphagia secondary to cricopharyngeal muscle dysfunction. Arch Otolaryngol 101:726-729, 1975.
19. Gay I, Chisin R, Elidan J. Myotomy of the cricopharyngeal muscle: A treatment for dysphagia and aspiration in neurological disorders. Rev Laryngol 105:271-274, 1984.
20. Bonavena L, Khan NA, DeMeester TR. Pharyngoesophageal dysfunctions: The role of cricopharyngeal myotomy. Arch Surg 120:541-549, 1985.
21. Millar H. The cervical treatment of cervical oesophageal and laryngo-pharyngeal dysphagia. Aust N Z J Surg 42:368-373, 1973.
22. Chodosh PL. Cricopharyngeal myotomy in the treatment of dysphagia. Laryngoscope 85:1862-1873, 1975.
23. Mitchell RL, Armanini GB. Cricopharyngeal myotomy: Treatment of dysphagia. Ann Surg 181:262-266, 1975.
24. Leonard JR, Smith H. Cricopharyngeal achalasia. Ann Otol Rhinol 79:907-910, 1970.
25. Orringer MB. Extended cervical esophago-myotomy for cricopharyngeal dysfunction. J Thorac Cardiovasc Surg 80:669-678, 1980.
26. Logemann JA. Swallowing physiology and pathophysiology. Otolaryngol Clin North Am 21:613-623, 1988.
27. Loizou LA, Small M, Dalton GA. Cricopharyngeal myotomy in motor neuron disease. J Neurol Neurosurg Psychiatry 43:42-45, 1980.
28. Lebo CP, Kwei Sang U, Norris FH. Cricopharyngeal myotomy in amyotrophic lateral sclerosis. Trans Pacific Coast Oto-Ophthal Soc 56:125-133, 1975.
29. Lebo CP, Kwei Sang U, Norris FH. Cricopharyngeal myotomy in amyotrophic lateral sclerosis. Laryngoscope 86:862-868, 1976.
30. Calne DB, Shaw DG, Spiers ASD, Stern GM. Swallowing in parkinsonism. Br J Radiol 43:456-457, 1970.
31. Akl BF, Blakeley WR. Late assessment of results of cricopharyngeal myotomy for cervical dysphagia. Am J Surg 128:818-822, 1974.
32. Henderson RD, Boszko A, Van Nostrand AWP, Pearson FG. Pharyngoesophageal dysphagia and recurrent laryngeal nerve palsy. J Thorac Cardiovasc Surg 68:507-512, 1977.
33. Mills CP. Dysphagia in progressive bulbar palsy relieved by division of the cricopharyngeus. J Laryngol Otol 78:963-964, 1964.
34. Bofenkamp B. The surgical correction of aphagia following bulbar poliomyelitis. Arch Otolaryngol 68:165-172, 1958.
35. Schneider MA, Nagourney J. Progressive supranuclear ophthalmoplegia association with cricopharyngeal dysfunction and recurrent pneumonia. JAMA 237:994-995, 1977.
36. Kaplan S. Paralysis of deglutition, a post poliomyelitis complication treated by section of the cricopharyngeus muscle. Ann Surg 133:572-576, 1951.
37. Nanson EM. Achalasia of cricopharyngeus muscle and pharyngeal diverticulum. Aust N Z J Med 80:41-48, 1974.
38. Wiles CM. Neurogenic dysphagia. J Neurol Neurosurg Psychiatry 54:1037-1039, 1991.

11

Surgical Management of Leiomyoma and Extramucosal Cysts of the Esophagus

Luigi Bonavina, M.D. • *Andrea Segalin, M.D.*
Raffaello Incarbone, M.D. • *Alberto Peracchia, M.D.*

Leiomyoma and extramucosal cysts represent the most common benign masses of the esophagus. Although leiomyomas occur five times more frequently than extramucosal cysts,[1] it is worthwhile to consider these conditions together because they are usually submucosal and present similar problems with diagnosis and surgical therapy.

Leiomyomas are smooth muscle cell tumors located in the lower or middle third of the esophagus. Only approximately 10% are found in the upper esophagus. The tumor is usually a solitary, encapsulated, round to oval mass between 2 and 5 cm in diameter. Occasionally, it is horseshoe-shaped or circumferential. Multiple tumors and leiomyomatosis of the esophagogastric junction are uncommon. Tumor growth is slow. A giant leiomyoma can cause ulceration of the overlying mucosa and possible bleeding. Reports describing sarcomatous degeneration are anecdotal.[2]

Extramucosal cysts are congenital lesions of mixed embryogenesis and their classification is controversial. They are usually classified as being either gastroenteric, bronchogenic, or esophageal reduplication cysts. The bronchogenic type occurs most frequently and is characterized by a lining of ciliated columnar epithelium and by the presence of cartilage. The prevailing site of these malformations is the posteroinferior mediastinum. Extramucosal cysts of the esophagus can be complicated by intracystic hemorrhage, perforation, or infection. Malignant degeneration has also been reported.[3]

Almost one half of the patients with leiomyoma and approximately one third of those with extramucosal cysts are asymptomatic. The diagnosis of a submucosal mass can be incidental, although some patients complain of nonspecific symptoms such as chest pain and dyspepsia. Dysphagia is more common in patients with leiomyoma.

Modern imaging techniques, such as computed tomography (CT) and endoscopic ultrasonography (EUS), allow an accurate evaluation of these lesions, although the differential diagnosis may be difficult in some circumstances. The indications for surgical therapy have often been questioned because of the absence or paucity of symptoms in some patients, the usually benign natural history of the disease, and the trauma of thoracotomy, which seems disproportionate to a relatively simple operation. Moreover, very little information exists about late results of surgery.

PATIENTS AND METHODS

Between 1967 and 1994, 66 patients with leiomyoma (group 1) and 11 patients with an extramucosal cyst of the esophagus (group 2) were treated.

Group 1 consisted of 53 men and 13 women (ratio 4:1), with a mean age of 46 years (range, 19 to 71 years). The main presenting symptoms were dysphagia in 35 patients (53%), heartburn and/or regurgitation in 11 patients (17%), and retrosternal pain in 10 patients (15%). Of the remaining 10 patients (15%), eight were asymptomatic and two had previous episodes of upper gastrointestinal bleeding from acute erosive gastritis or an active duodenal ulcer. Preoperative workup included a barium swallow study and upper gastrointestinal endoscopy in all patients. Six patients had previously undergone endoscopic biopsy of the leiomyoma elsewhere. CT scan and/or EUS were performed in the last 22 patients. Esophageal manometry and/or 24-hour esophageal pH monitoring were performed only in selected patients who had concomitant esophageal disorders.

Group 2 consisted of six women and five men (ratio 1.2:1), with a mean age of 40 years (range, 16 to 53 years). Eight patients were symptomatic and complained of retrosternal or epigastric pain. Three of them also had mild dysphagia for solid food. The remaining three patients (27%) were asymptomatic and the mass was discovered incidentally on a routine chest radiograph.

The diagnostic workup included a chest radiograph, barium swallow study, esophagoscopy, CT scan, and more recently EUS. In two patients with a long-lasting history of heartburn unresponsive to medical therapy, esophageal manometry, 24-hour pH monitoring, and esophageal transit scintigraphy were performed.

RESULTS
Group 1

The leiomyoma was located in the middle third of the thoracic esophagus in 36 patients (55%), in the lower third in 16 patients (24%), in the upper third in 10 patients (15%), and at the gastroesophageal junction in four patients (6%). Associated esophageal disorders were found in 19 patients. Fifteen patients (23%) had a hiatal hernia, four patients (6%) had epiphrenic diverticulum, and three patients (5%) had achalasia. Erosive esophagitis was documented in three patients with hiatal hernia.

The operation consisted of simple tumor enucleation in 63 patients. The procedure was initially performed through a conventional surgical approach in 55 patients. A right thoracotomy was used in 42 cases, a left thoracotomy in five cases, and a laparotomy in five cases. A right thoracoscopic approach was attempted in the last eight patients and the enucleation was successfully completed in six cases using a four-port technique. Video esophagoscopy was routinely performed to assist the thoracoscopic procedure with the aim to verify mucosal integrity, step by step, from inside the lumen.

An additional surgical procedure was synchronously performed during thoracotomy or laparotomy in 10 patients with concomitant disorders. Nissen fundoplication was performed in three patients, Heller myotomy with Dor fundoplication in three patients, diverticulectomy with myotomy and modified Belsey fundoplication in two patients, and simple diverticulectomy in two patients.

The size of the enucleated tumor ranged between 2 and 10 cm. Five were horseshoe-shaped tumors. In three patients, multiple adjacent tumors were found. The muscular layer of the esophagus was approximated in all but two patients. In the first patient, after enucleation of a 10×8 cm leiomyoma, the defect was too large to allow a tension-free suture. Vicryl mesh was therefore used to prevent mucosal bulging. In the second patient, who was operated on through a thoracoscopic approach, the muscle was not approximated because of technical difficulties in suturing.

In three patients, two women with a diffuse leiomyomatosis of the distal esophagus and a man with a huge leiomyoma at the esophagogastric junction, an esophageal resection was performed. The alimentary tract continuity was reestablished by means of intrathoracic esophagogastrostomy at the apex of the chest in two patients and intrathoracic left colon interposition in one patient.

In all patients, histology showed the typical features of interlaced bundles of smooth muscle cells with absent mitoses and hypovascularity. Diffuse leiomyomatosis was characterized by confluent nodular thickening of the esophagus and cardia combined with some degree of muscular hypertrophy.

There was no operative mortality. Complications of leiomyoma enucleation with the open procedure consisted of an intraoperative mucosal tear in seven patients. Esophageal perforation was more common in patients who had previous endoscopic biopsy (three of six patients [50%]) than in those who had not (four of 49 patients [8.1%]; $p < 0.01$). All mucosal lesions were repaired without consequence using 4-0 Vicryl sutures. One patient required emergency thoracotomy because of bleeding from an intercostal vessel. In one patient, an esophagopleural leak developed on the third postoperative day, requiring reoperation and mucosal repair.

The thoracoscopic approach was converted to a formal thoracotomy in two patients because of the inability to exclude the lung in one patient who had a large mediastinal goiter and because of a mucosal tear in the other patient in whom no preoperative biopsy had been performed. One patient in whom the muscle layer had not been approximated complained of persistent, intractable dysphagia. A barium swallow study showed a pseudodiverticular mucosal bulging in the middle third of the esophagus at the level of the enucleation site. Esophageal manometry demonstrated an area of segmental aperistalsis beginning 29 cm from the nostrils and extending for a length of approximately 5 cm. Reoperation through a right thoracotomy was performed a few months later and consisted of simple approximation of the muscle edges. Dysphagia resolved and the radiologic and manometric abnormalities disappeared.

Complications of esophageal resection included gastric outlet obstruction requiring pyloromyotomy in one patient after a gastric pull-up and stricture of the esophagocolic anastomosis requiring multiple dilations.

The median follow-up time was 53 months (range, 12 to 248 months). No recurrence of leiomyoma was observed. Overall, seven patients (11%) complained of heartburn and/or epigastric pain responsive to H_2 blockers or omeprazole. Four of those patients had symptoms related to gastroesophageal reflux or duodenal ulcer prior to the operation. One of these patients had a hiatal hernia and abnormal gastroesophageal reflux with erosive esophagitis diagnosed before undergoing thoracoscopic enucleation of a leiomyoma of the upper third of the esophagus and was successfully treated with a laparoscopic Nissen-Rossetti fundoplication a few months later.

In two patients the reflux symptoms appeared after resection of an epiphrenic diverticulum, myotomy, and partial fundoplication and in one patient after simple enucleation of a middle third leiomyoma. Twenty-four–hour esophageal pH monitoring showed an abnormal esophageal acid exposure in these three patients who are currently being treated with H_2 blockers.

No late complications developed during a follow-up time of 9 to 15 years in the three patients who underwent esophageal resection.

Group 2

The mass was located in the posteroinferior mediastinum in 10 patients and in the upper mediastinum in one patient. In all patients, an extrinsic compression with intact mucosa was evident on barium swallow examination. In the two patients who complained of heartburn, the results of esophageal manometry and 24-hour pH monitoring were normal. The esophageal transit scintigraphy showed delayed clearance of the radionuclide in the proximal two thirds of the esophagus.

A preoperative diagnosis of extramucosal cyst was quite obvious in five of the seven patients who were investigated by EUS and CT scan. In the other two patients, and in two additional patients who underwent CT scan alone, the findings suggested the diagnosis of leiomyoma because of the high density of the cyst contents.

All patients underwent surgical excision of the mass. A posterolateral thoracotomy was used in 10 patients and a thoracoscopy was used in the last patient. According to the site of the mass, six patients underwent left thoracotomy, four patients underwent right thoracotomy, and one patient underwent right thoracoscopy using a three-port technique. In all patients the cyst was enucleated without opening the esophageal mucosa. The muscle layers of the esophagus were bluntly dissected and the edges were approximated by interrupted sutures after removal of the cyst. Only one cyst was external but it was still adjacent to the esophageal wall.

The diameter of the cysts ranged from 2 to 4.5 cm and most contained a clear, jelly-like fluid. Histologic examination showed an epithelial lining of the ciliated columnar type covered by smooth muscle that was often infiltrated by chronic inflammatory cells. Cartilage was present in the cyst, which was external to the esophageal wall.

No postoperative morbidity was recorded. Nine patients were asymptomatic at a median follow-up time of 2.3 years (range, 13 to 77 months). One patient complained of dyspepsia and occasional regurgitation and vomiting. A barium esophagogram showed a pseudodiverticular defect in the distal esophagus corresponding to the site of the excised cyst. No esophagitis was found on endoscopy. Twenty-four–hour esophageal pH monitoring showed an abnormal esophageal acid exposure. Radionuclide examination demonstrated markedly delayed gastric emptying. The patient was treated with H_2 blockers and cisapride with satisfactory results. Another patient complained of persistent dyspepsia. Antral gastritis with *Helicobacter pylori* infection was found on endoscopy and the patient was successfully treated with omeprazole.

DISCUSSION

The results of this study show that the diagnosis of leiomyoma and extramucosal cyst of the esophagus was incidental in 12% and 27% of the patients, respectively. Dysphagia was far more common in patients with leiomyoma.

Once a submucosal mass of the esophagus is suspected on the chest radiograph or the barium swallow examination, endoscopy should be performed to evaluate the mucosa. If the mucosa overlying the mass is normal, no biopsies should be taken because they would complicate surgical removal. In our series, the incidence of intraoperative esophageal perforation was significantly greater in patients with leiomyoma who had previously undergone endoscopic biopsy. Parendoscopic needle biopsy of paraesophageal cysts has been reported,[4] but we believe that the aspirate does not provide useful information and the procedure has the potential of infecting the mass.

Modern imaging techniques are quite reliable for excluding malignancy in patients presenting with an extramucosal mass of the esophagus. Cancer was not suspected in any of our patients. However, the differential diagnosis between leiomyoma and extramucosal cyst was not always obvious because of the high density of the cyst contents. It has been shown that mucinous cysts may present with fine internal echoes simulating leiomyoma, but with strong acoustic enhancement.[5] Finally, imaging techniques may help in the evaluation of the topographic relationships of these masses so that the most appropriate surgical approach can be planned.

The usual clinical course of leiomyomas and extramucosal cysts is benign and many patients may remain asymptomatic. The indications for surgical therapy are based on the presence of symptoms, the size of the mass, the inability to exclude a malignancy, and the presence of concomitant disease requiring treatment, such as achalasia or hiatal hernia. Simple endosonographic follow-up has been advocated for leiomyomas of less than 3 cm in diameter with an echo-homogeneous pattern and smooth margins.[6] Conversely, all presumed cysts should be resected because an operation can be hazardous when the cyst becomes symptomatic and because a definitive diagnosis can be established only on the surgical specimen. Cyst aspiration has been proposed as an alternative to operation, but this method is not recommended because of the risk of cyst recurrence, which carries a significant morbidity.[7]

Surgical enucleation is the treatment of choice for submucosal masses of the esophagus. An accurate preoperative evaluation is mandatory in these patients to precisely assess the position of the mass and the clinical relevance of associated esophageal disorders, which may require a change in surgical strategy.

The conventional surgical approach consists of enucleation of the mass after splitting the overlying muscle layer. Both vagal nerves should be identified and preserved. A plane can easily be found between the mass and the esophageal mucosa, unless there is inflammation or mucosal damage following endoscopic biopsy. Mucosal integrity should be evaluated using air insufflation through the nasogastric tube after surgical dissection.

We emphasize the need to approximate the muscle edges of the esophagus after enucleation of the mass. A pseudodiverticulum has occurred twice in our experience and may appear in an area of disorganized muscular anatomy, causing defective propulsive activity of the esophagus and symptoms. This impression is supported by the immediate restoration of esophageal transit and the reversal of the manometric abnormalities documented in our patient who underwent thoracotomy and reconstruction of the muscle layer following thoracoscopic enucleation of a leiomyoma.

The conventional approach through a formal thoracotomy has the potential of causing excessive postoperative pain and discomfort to the patient. Moreover, the hospital stay and the recovery period are prolonged. Recent advances in minimally invasive surgery have led to a less traumatic approach to benign esophageal disorders. Leiomyoma and extramucosal cysts represent an excellent indication for video-assisted thoracoscopic enucleation, and the feasibility and the satisfactory early clinical results of this approach have been clearly documented.[8,9] The videothoracoscopic approach is as effective and safe as in open surgery and has the advantage of providing a superb and magnified vision of the operative field, thus reducing postoperative discomfort and improving the cosmetic result of the operation. However, the procedure should only be performed by thoracic surgeons trained in open surgery and in advanced thoracoscopic techniques.

During thoracoscopic enucleation, permanent transillumination through the esophagoscope is very useful because it allows step-by-step control of the integrity of the esophageal mucosa. Esophagoscopy allows air inflation and deflation of the esophageal lumen, making it easier to identify the border between the mucosa and the leiomyoma.

Follow-up of the patients is mandatory after removal of leiomyoma or extramucosal cysts, especially in patients with previous history of gastroesophageal reflux disease (GERD). It has been postulated that the incidence of esophagitis can increase after excision of the mass because of a decreased propulsive activity of the esophagus and impairment of the acid-clearing mechanism.[10] Suturing the muscle edges after excision of a submucosal mass of the esophagus may improve the long-term outcome of the operation by preserving the propulsive activity of the esophageal body.

REFERENCES

1. Payne WS, Olsen AM. The Esophagus. Philadelphia: Lea & Febiger, 1974.
2. Postlethwait RW. Surgery of the Esophagus. Norwalk, Conn.: Appleton-Century-Crofts, 1986.
3. Enterline H, Thompson J. Pathology of the Esophagus. New York: Springer-Verlag, 1984.
4. Kuhlman J, Fishman K, Wang K, et al. Esophageal duplication cyst: CT and transesophageal needle aspiration. AJR 145:531-532, 1985.
5. Bondestam S, Salo J, Salonen O, et al. Imaging of congenital esophageal cysts in adults. Gastrointest Radiol 15:279-281, 1990.
6. Rosch T, Lorenz R, Dancygier H, et al. Endosonographic diagnosis of submucosal upper gastrointestinal tract tumor. Scand J Gastroenterol 27:1-8, 1992.
7. St-Georges R, Deslauriers J, Duranceau A, et al. Clinical spectrum of bronchogenic cysts of the mediastinum and lung in the adult. Ann Thorac Surg 52:6-13, 1991.
8. Bardini R, Segalin A, Ruol A, et al. Videothoracoscopic enucleation of esophageal leiomyoma. Ann Thorac Surg 54:576-577, 1992.
9. Mouroux J, Bourgeon A, Benchimal D, et al. Les kistes bronchogeniques de l'oesophage. Chirurgie traditionnelle ou video-chirurgie? Chirurgie 117:564-568, 1991.
10. Ala-Kulju K, Salo J. Smooth muscle tumours of the oesophagus. Scand J Thorac Cardiovasc Surg 21:65-68, 1987.

12

Therapeutic Endoscopy of Benign Esophageal Diseases

Andrea Segalin, M.D. • *Luigi Bonavina, M.D.*

Therapeutic endoscopy of benign esophageal diseases includes endoscopic management of Zenker's diverticulum and achalasia, dilation of strictures, removal of foreign bodies, and ablation of Barrett's epithelium. Intraoperative endoscopy is now routinely used in association with several surgical procedures performed through a laparoscopic or thoracoscopic approach.

At present, a variety of complementary or competitive procedures such as bougienage, balloon dilation, and laser treatment are available. However, the optimal treatment is often achieved with the integration of all endoscopic options related to the general conditions, stage of the disease, and surgical risk of each patient. Operative endoscopy of the esophagus does not represent an alternative to surgery and should be performed in a department where surgical facilities and expertise are promptly available.

DIVISION OF THE SEPTUM IN ZENKER'S DIVERTICULUM

An endoscopic treatment of the hypopharyngeal diverticulum was proposed early this century[1] in the section of the septum between the diverticulum and the esophagus. The common wall includes the upper esophageal sphincter. This procedure has been performed for many years by means of rigid endoscopy and diathermy or laser.[2] Nevertheless, the operative time of this technique is long and the procedure still entails a relatively high morbidity rate, which is represented mainly by bleeding, leak, and mediastinitis.

The use of a Weerda diverticuloscope (Karl Storz, Tuttlingen, Germany) and a modified Endo GIA stapler has recently been proposed.[3,4] Stapling of the septum is an innovative procedure that appears simpler, faster, and safer than electrocoagulation or laser. With a single or double application of the Endo GIA stapler, the posterior esophageal wall is sutured to the wall of the diverticulum for a length of 30 or 60 mm and the tissue is transected between the two triple-staggered staple rows. The procedure, which requires a few minutes, is performed under general anesthesia with nasotracheal intubation. A complete section of the septum to include the length of the diverticulum has been made possible by a modification of the stapler. A shortened distal port is used to insert into the diverticulum.

This procedure is contraindicated in patients with a small diverticulum (3 cm or less) in whom it is impossible to include the whole length of the upper esophageal sphincter in the stapler. This approach can also prove difficult in patients with cervical osteoarthritis, because of the inability to extend the neck, and in those with a reduced opening capacity of the mouth, because of the limited access of the instruments.

DILATION OF ACHALASIA

The choice between an endoscopic treatment and surgical cardiomyotomy as initial treatment of achalasia is still controversial and depends mainly on the stage of disease, the physician's aggressiveness, and the patient's attitude.

Several studies have suggested that a treatment regimen beginning with dilation is usually effective and has a shorter recovery and less overall cost than initial cardiomyotomy.[5,6] The success and the morbidity rates of pneumatic dilation reported in different series depend on the technical characteristics and diameter of the balloon and on the experience of the endoscopist. Generally, long-term results of endoscopic dilation are generally inferior to those of surgery in young patients and in patients with recurrent achalasia after a first dilation.[5] Moreover, cardiomyotomy may be technically more difficult after endoscopic dilation because of fibrosis of the muscular layers that usually follows forced pneumatic dilation. At present, pneumatic dilation can be performed as initial treatment of achalasia in old patients in poor general condition and at high surgical risk.[7]

Endoscopy can be performed without any preparation only in patients with grade I disease. When the esophageal diameter is noted to be increased on the radiologic study, a nasoesophageal tube must be placed for 24 hours to allow an adequate washout of residual ingesta. The procedure is generally performed with conscious sedation, which can be obtained with intravenous administration of midazolam, diazepam, or propofol. A higher prevalence of perforation has been reported in series in which dilation was performed under general anesthesia.[8] Premedication with atropine or hyoscine butylbromide may reduce the lower esophageal sphincter (LES) pressure, increase the compliance of the cardia to the balloon, and reduce the effectiveness of the procedure.

Of the several dilators that are available, the Rigiflex balloon (Microvasive, Watertown, Mass.) is recommended. The main characteristic of this dilator is its low compliance so that inflation is restricted to its designed diameter (30, 35, and 40 mm). In contrast, the final diameter of many other devices depends on the inflation pressure, which may significantly increase the risk of perforation. The Rigiflex dilator is inserted over a guidewire, which may prove useful to place the balloon across the cardia in patients with a markedly dilated esophagus. Nevertheless, in patients with a tortuous sigmoid esophagus, the insertion of the dilator in the correct position can still be difficult. In such circumstances, the use of a rigid overtube to straighten the esophagus and allow access to the gastroesophageal junction may be helpful.[9] During dilation the correct position of the dilator must be controlled with fluoroscopy or an endoscope inserted beside the catheter with the tip proximal to the transparent balloon. This latter solution is preferable because it allows the operator to control the mucosa of the gastric cardia during dilation in real time. Therefore, any minimal mucosal lesion can be immediately recognized by direct vision or by the presence of blood. Even a modest bleeding during the inflation of the balloon must be regarded as a sign of imminent esophageal perforation requiring immediate deflation of the dilator. The choice of the diameter of the balloon for the first dilation depends on the size of the patient and the stage of the disease. Progressive dilation under endoscopic control is always recommended. In small patients with early disease and a LES resting pressure lower than 25 mm Hg, a 30 mm balloon can be used initially. The 35 mm balloon is usually employed in all other patients. Once the dilator is in the correct position, the pressure must be gradually increased to 10 psi and maintained for 1 minute. The dilator is deflated, pushed into the stomach, and the cardia region is carefully inspected with the endoscope. The balloon is repositioned and inflated to 15 or 20 psi according to the patient's compliance and endoscopic findings and maintained for another minute. A good functional result is usually evident at the end of the procedure when the gastroesophageal junction appears to be open. When the endoscopic appearance of the cardia is not satisfactory, a further dilation with the same or a larger balloon should be performed during the same endoscopic session. An esophagogram with water-soluble contrast is usually performed within 24 hours to evaluate the passage of the contrast media across the cardia and the presence of the gastric air pocket. The patient is discharged on H_2-blocker therapy for 3 weeks to prevent damage from reflux. Manometry is performed 1 month later.

Esophageal perforation is the main complication of forced pneumatic dilation. If minimal bleeding occurs, the dilator must be immediately deflated, removed, and the mucosa washed and inspected. In the presence of an intraparietal mucosal lesion, a double-lumen nasogastric tube must be positioned under endoscopic control. An esophagogram with water-soluble contrast should be performed immediately and medical therapy with antibiotics, H_2 blockers, nasogastric aspiration, and parenteral nutrition should be begun. Conservative treatment of perforation after pneumatic dilation is usually effective if the lesion is recognized immediately and promptly managed.[10] Surgery is required in patients with full-thickness and larger lesions, significant bleeding, or peritonitis.

The endoscopic injection of the toxin of *Clostridium botulinum* in the LES has been introduced recently in the management of achalasia.[11] The rationale for this treatment is because of the specific anticholinergic effect of the toxin, which allows a significant decrease of the sphincter resting pressure. Although promising results have been reported without major side effects, this technique must be validated by larger series with a longer follow-up and must still be regarded as investigational.

BENIGN ESOPHAGEAL STRICTURE

Endoscopic dilation is the mainstay in the treatment of benign esophageal strictures following chronic reflux esophagitis, surgical anastomosis, variceal sclerotherapy, webs, and caustic injuries. At present, most of these strictures can be treated endoscopically in the first instance.[12]

In patients with stricture from reflux esophagitis, an antireflux repair is indicated after proper dilation to avoid lifelong dilation and medication. Esophageal resection is still the treatment of choice for long strictures in patients with reflux or caustic ingestion or in the presence of Barrett's esophagus with severe dysplasia.[13]

The technique of endoscopic dilation depends on the radiologic and endoscopic characteristics of the stricture rather than its etiology.[14] Mercury-filled Maloney bougies were initially used for almost all esophageal strictures. Although this technique is still widely used, especially in the United States, it is suitable only for straight and relatively soft strictures.[15] Dilation over a guidewire through a scope has almost completely replaced the use of Maloney dilators, especially in Europe. The advantage of endoscopic dilation is that an appropriate evaluation of the diameter and the characteristics, including histology, of the stricture can be made before and after dilation. In addition, complex, tight, and angulated strictures can also be treated.[16]

The procedure is usually performed under local pharyngeal anesthesia and conscious sedation with intravenous administration of midazolam, diazepam, or propofol. General anesthesia should be avoided because it is important to evaluate the patient's reactions during the procedure. Antibiotic prophylaxis is indicated in high-risk patients or in the presence of prosthetic heart valves and vascular shunts. Preoperative evaluation of the stricture with barium swallow is mandatory. It is also advisable to use fluoroscopy to aid in the placement of the guidewire in long and angulated strictures, which are difficult to pass blindly. The use of a pediatric instrument of 7.9 mm diameter (Olympus GIF-XP20, Pentax FG-24X) or an ultraslim instrument of 5.2 mm diameter (Olympus GIF-N30) allows the successful management of almost all cases. A larger instrument with a channel of at least 2.8 mm diameter (Olympus GIF-PQ20) must be used when a pneumatic dilation is planned.

The over-the-wire bougies available are Eder-Puestow (Key-Med), Savary-Gillard (Wilson Cook), and American Endoscopy (Bard). The Eder-Puestow olives are more traumatic than the other polyvinyl tubes. Nevertheless, because they are rigid, their use may still be required as the last resort when all the other endoscopic options fail. The Savary-Gillard dilators have become very popular because they allow a less traumatic dilation and are better tolerated by the patient. They have a radiopaque band at the point of maximum diameter, which assists with their use under fluoroscopy. American Endoscopy bougies are impregnated with barium sulfate, which makes them clearly visible at fluoroscopy, and they are more rigid and have a shortened tip. All of these dilators are of the "push type," which exert both axial and radial forces on the stricture. Pneumatic balloon dilators exert the entire dilating force radially and simultaneously over the entire length of the stenotic segment.[17,18] Theoretically, this should allow a safer and more efficient dilation. The noncompliant balloon material ensures that the maximum inflation diameter is achieved and maintained through a wide range of inflation pressures. The balloons must be inflated with water, which allows a faster and more effective inflation of the balloon to its final diameter. The maximal inflation pressure ranges between 25 and 50 psi according to the diameter of the balloon. For fibrotic and tight strictures a new high-pressure noncompliant dilator is available (Max Force, Microvasive), which can be inflated up to 150 psi (10 ATM). At present, the two types of balloon dilators available are through-the-scope (TTS) (Microvasive, Bard) and over-the-wire (OTW) balloon (Microvasive). The TTS type is introduced through the operative channel of the instrument and allows dilation with real-time endoscopic control. Angulated and tortuous strictures in which the passage of the deflated dilator is difficult or impossible limit its use. The OTW balloon dilator is similar to the TTS, but it is provided with a central channel for a guidewire that is passed through the stricture. To ensure a safe dilation the guidewire should be placed under direct vision in the antrum for dilation of strictures of the thoracic esophagus and in the duodenum for dilation of cardiac strictures. The external part of the guidewire is entrusted to a nurse assistant who is trained to ensure that the wire is kept constantly in place and not allowed to slip in or out. In addition it must be kept taut at the time of dilation to avoid kinking the wire itself and the dilator. If the stricture is too narrow to permit the passage even of the pediatric or ultraslim endoscope, the endoscopist has the choice of either proceeding with the help of fluoroscopy or using a TTS balloon. The TTS balloon is used for straight strictures and requires an endoscope with an operating channel of at least 2.8 mm of diameter. The passage of the guidewire blindly through the stricture under fluoroscopic control is usually safe and easy. Nevertheless, in patients with extremely angulated strictures, especially after esophagovisceral anastomosis, the placement of a traditional guidewire may prove impossible. In these patients, intraoperative radiologic identification of the stricture must be obtained by injecting some contrast media through a catheter inserted through the endoscope. Immediately after the contrast injection, the placement of a biliary J-tip wire with a torque-vise at its proximal extremity may be attempted. The biliary wire is soft, has a coated surface, and can be passed through extremely tortuous strictures.

The diameter of the first dilator should be just bigger than the estimated diameter of the stricture. With experience the operator learns to appreciate the "feel" of the passage through a strictured area. The "rule of three" is recommended when a number of dilators are used at a single session. The first dilator that meets with resistance determines the stricture size and no more than three successively larger dilators (with increments of 1 mm or 3 F) should be used. After removal of the last dilator along with the guidewire, an endoscopic review of the stricture is recommended.

Complications of dilation may be related to anatomic abnormalities, to the guidewire, and to the technique itself. Anatomic abnormalities, such as the presence of hiatal hernia or diverticula, or irregular eccentric strictures, which may interfere with the proper placement of the guidewire, should be evaluated by preoperative esophagogram. The risk of perforation related to the blind placement of the guidewire is greater without the use of fluoroscopy and in patients with recent caustic strictures.[19] The most common cause of perforation is overdilation and occurs more frequently with Savary-Gillard bougies and the pneumatic dilator. The feel of a resistance is not very reliable when using these dilators and the tightness of the stricture is often underestimated. It is therefore important to closely follow the "rule of three."

Identification of high-risk strictures is mandatory to reduce the morbidity by the use of fluoroscopy.[20] Whatever the cause of perforation, it is important to recognize this complication early because morbidity and mortality are increased by a delayed diagnosis. Endoscopic evaluation of the stricture at the conclusion of the dilation allows prompt identification of a mucosal defect. A contrast esophagogram with water-soluble contrast should be performed immediately when perforation is suspected.

ESOPHAGEAL WEBS

Esophageal web is a relatively uncommon cause of intermittent dysphagia to solids. Radiologic and endoscopic findings of a diaphragm are usually characteristic. Endoscopic dilation is the treatment of choice in these patients. This is the only occasion in which a large-size dilator can be introduced without first passing smaller dilators.[12] A high success rate is reported by the use of a single endoscopic dilation performed independently of the technique or the dilator. Maloney, Savary-Gillard, and pneumatic dilators have been used with comparable results. The only important factor is the size of the dilator, which should not be smaller than 45 or 50 F. In a small subset of patients who fail to respond to standard esophageal dilation, endoscopic incision of the stricture can be successfully performed by means of diathermy or Nd:YAG laser.[21]

REMOVAL OF FOREIGN BODIES

Removal of impacted esophageal foreign bodies has usually been performed by means of rigid endoscopy under general anesthesia. Flexible fiberoptic endoscopes with multiple large-size operative channels (Olympus GIF-2T200) and dedicated forceps have simplified the management of these patients. With conscious sedation, foreign bodies can be removed with a high success rate and a negligible morbidity and mortality.[22] Cost is low when compared with rigid esophagoscopy. Sharp and pointed foreign bodies require the use of a protector hood to place onto the tip of the instrument or an overtube to improve the safety of the procedure.[23] When a double-channel instrument is not available, the simultaneous use of two flexible endoscopes has been also reported.[24] Although a higher success rate for the removal of foreign bodies is still reported for rigid esophagoscopy, a higher complication rate is to be expected. The flexible fiberoptic endoscopic technique is therefore attempted first.[22] If flexible esophagoscopy proves unsuccessful, rigid esophagoscopy with general anesthesia should be performed.

LASER PHOTOABLATION OF BARRETT'S EPITHELIUM

Barrett's esophagus is widely regarded as a risk factor for adenocarcinoma of the esophagus.[25] Theoretically, regression of Barrett's epithelium might prevent the development of dysplasia and cancer. Regression of the metaplastic epithelium has been reported only sporadically with omeprazole or antireflux surgery. For these reasons, ablation of Barrett's epithelium with endoscopic laser therapy has been proposed in addition to acid suppression. Both Nd:YAG and argon dye lasers and photodynamic therapy have been used with promising results.[26-28] At present, these reports should be regarded as investigational. Further studies with long-term follow-up are needed to assess the role of this treatment in patients with Barrett's esophagus.

INTRAOPERATIVE ENDOSCOPY IN MINIMALLY INVASIVE SURGERY

Several surgical procedures on the esophagus have recently been performed through a minimally invasive approach.[29] The laparoscopic or the thoracoscopic approach has proved to be less traumatic than traditional open surgery, allowing procedures to be performed in patients with achalasia, leiomyoma, diverticula, and gastroesophageal reflux. Moreover, the view of the operative field is magnified by the camera. Nevertheless, the bidimensional view and the lack of tactile perception may increase the difficulty of some surgical maneuvers.

During thoracoscopic enucleation of esophageal leiomyoma, intraoperative endoscopy allows a prompt localization of the tumor. The surgical maneuvers are clearly seen from inside the esophagus, and this can be helpful in maintaining the dissection in the layer between the mucosa and the leiomyoma. Moreover, the integrity of the mucosa can be continuously verified and any minimal tear can be immediately recognized by air leakage in the operative field.[30]

When a thoracoscopic approach is planned in patients with epiphrenic diverticula, associated with an abnormally high basal pressure of the LES, incoordination, or incomplete relaxation, a preoperative pneumatic dilation with a Rigiflex balloon 30 mm of diameter inflated at 10 psi for 1 minute can be performed.[31] Intraoperatively, endoscopy is performed to inflate, deflate, and transilluminate the diverticulum to make the identification and dissection easier. Any mucosal lesion can be promptly identified from inside the esophagus because of air leakage in the operative field. Diverticulectomy is performed by Endo GIA, and the residual lumen of the esophagus is verified and calibrated from inside by the endoscope avoiding the risk of an excessive mucosal resection and consequent stenosis. At the end of the procedure, the esophagus is inflated and the operative field is immersed in saline solution to verify the integrity of the staple line.

Esophagomyotomy of the LES in patients with achalasia can be successfully performed through a thoracoscopic or laparoscopic approach. Intraoperative endoscopy assists the procedure by distending the gastroesophageal junction with a Rigiflex dilator of 30 mm of diameter, which is inflated and deflated alternatively at a pressure that must not exceed 1 to 2 psi. In this way, the esophageal mucosa at the level of the cardia is displayed and can be easily dissected from the muscular layers. Before performing the antireflux Dor procedure, the esophageal lumen can be inflated and the myotomy site checked endoscopically.

In patients with gastroesophageal reflux disease intraoperative endoscopy can be helpful only in selected cases to facilitate the identification and the dissection of the gastroesophageal junction.

REFERENCES

1. Mosher H. Webs and pouches of the esophagus, their diagnosis and treatment. Surg Gynecol Obstet 25:175-187, 1917.
2. Dohlman G, Mattson O. The endoscopic operation for hypopharyngeal diverticula. Arch Otolaryngol 71:744-752, 1960.
3. Narne S, Bonavina L, Guido E, Peracchia A. Treatment of Zenker's diverticulum by endoscopic stapling. Endosurgery 1:118-180, 1993.
4. Collard J, Otte J, Kestens P. Endoscopic stapling technique of esophagodiverticulostomy for Zenker's diverticulum. Ann Thorac Surg 56:573-576, 1993.
5. Parkman HP, Reynolds JC, Ouyang A, Rosato EF, Eisenberg JM, Cohen S. Pneumatic dilatation or esophagomyotomy treatment for idiopathic achalasia: Clinical outcomes and cost analysis. Dig Dis Sci 38:75-85, 1993.
6. Kadakia SC, Wong RKH. Graded pneumatic dilatation using Rigiflex achalasia dilatators in patients with primary esophageal achalasia. Am J Gastroenterol 88:34-38, 1993.
7. Nair LA, Reynolds JC, Parkman HP, Ouyang A, Strom BL, Rosato EF, Cohen S. Complications during pneumatic dilatation for achalasia or diffuse esophageal spasm, early clinical characteristics and outcome. Dig Dis Sci 38:1893-1904, 1993.
8. Andersen LI, Frederiksen HJ, Lund JT, Sorensen HR. Balloon dilatation of the lower oesophageal sphincter. Eur J Surg 157:665-667, 1991.
9. Bernstein D, Barkin JS. Pneumatic dilatation of a sigmoid esophagus using an overtube. Gastrointest Endosc 39:549-550, 1993.
10. Schwartz HM, Cahow CE, Traube M. Outcome after perforation sustained during pneumatic dilatation for achalasia. Dig Dis Sci 38:1409-1413, 1993.
11. Pasricha PJ, Ravich WJ, Kalloo AN. Effects of intrasphincteric botulinum toxin on the lower esophageal sphincter in piglets. Gastroenterology 105:1045-1049, 1993.
12. Anand BS. Eder-Puestow and Savary dilators. Hepatogastroenterology 39:494-496, 1992.
13. Bonavina L, Fontebasso V, Bardini R, Baessato M, Peracchia A. Surgical treatment of reflux stricture of the esophagus. Br J Surg 80:317-320, 1993.
14. Pang-Chi Chen. Endoscopic balloon dilation of esophageal strictures following surgical anastomoses, endoscopic variceal sclerotherapy and corrosive investigation. Gastrointest Endosc 38:586-589, 1992.
15. Harrison ME, Sanowski RA. Mercury bougies dilatation of benign esophageal strictures. Hepatogastroenterology 39:497-501, 1992.
16. Neuhaus H. Esophageal therapeutic endoscopy, laser and prosthesis. Curr Opin Gastroenterol 10:473-480, 1994.
17. Saeed ZA. Balloon dilatation of benign esophageal stenosis. Hepatogastroenterology 39:490-493, 1992.
18. Abele JE. The physics of esophageal dilatation. Hepatogastroenterology 39:486-489, 1992.
19. Kadakia SC, Parker A, Carrougher JG, Shaffer RT. Esophageal dilatation with polyvinyl bougies using a marked guidewire without the aid of fluoroscopy: An update. Am J Gastroenterol 88:1381-1386, 1993.
20. Mohandas KM, Santhi Swaroop V, Desai DC. Marked wire-guided esophageal dilatation and the need of fluoroscopy. Gastrointest Endosc 38:634-635, 1992.
21. Burdick JS, Venu RP, Hogan WJ. Cutting the defiant lower esophageal ring. Gastrointest Endosc 39:616-619, 1993.
22. Berggreen PJ, Harrison ME, Sanowski RA, Ingebo K, Noland B, Zierer S. Techniques and complications of esophageal foreign body extraction in children and adults. Gastrointest Endosc 39:626-630, 1993.

23. Kelley JE, Leech MH, Carr MG. A safe and cost-effective protocol for the management of esophageal coins in children. J Pediatr Surg 28:898-900, 1993.
24. Bertoni G, Pacchione L, Sassatelli R, Ricci E, Mortilla MG, Gumina C. A new protector device for safe endoscopic removal of sharp gastroesophageal foreign bodies in infants. J Pediatr Gastroenterol Nutr 16:393-396, 1993.
25. Hameeteman W, Tytgat GNJ, Houthof HJ, van der Tweel JG. Barrett's esophagus: Development of dysplasia and adenocarcinoma. Gastroenterology 96:1249-1256, 1989.
26. Berenson MM, Johnson TD, Markowitz NR, Buchi KN, Samowitz WS. Restoration of squamous mucosa after ablation of Barrett's esophageal epithelium. Gastroenterology 104:1686-1691, 1993.
27. Sampliner RE, Hixson LJ, Fennerty MB, Garewal HS. Regression of Barrett's esophagus by laser ablation in an antiacid environment. Dig Dis Sci 38:365-368, 1993.
28. Laukka MA, Wang KK, Cameron AJ, Alexander GL. The use of photodynamic therapy in the treatment of Barrett's esophagus: Preliminary results. Gastrointest Endosc 39:A291, 1993.
29. Peracchia A, Segalin A, Bonavina L, Granelli P, Pavanello M, Rosati R. Intraoperative endoscopy for minimally invasive esophageal surgery. Endosurgery 2:53-55, 1994.
30. Bardini R, Segalin A, Ruol A, Pavanello M, Peracchia A. Thoracoscopic enucleation of esophageal leiomyoma. Ann Thorac Surg 54:576-577, 1992.
31. Peracchia A, Bonavina L, Rosati R, Bona S. Thoracoscopic resection of epiphrenic esophageal diverticula. In Peters JH, DeMeester TR, eds. Minimally Invasive Surgery of the Foregut. St. Louis: Quality Medical Publishing, 1994, pp 101-116.

13

Reoperation for Failed Antireflux Procedures

Simon Y.K. Law, F.R.C.S.(Ed) • *Jeffrey A. Hagen, M.D.*
Werner K.H. Kauer, M.D. • *Tom R. DeMeester, M.D.*

Surgery for gastroesophageal reflux disease (GERD) differs from most surgical procedures in that it is mechanistic rather than extirpative. As such, the focus of the procedure is on improving function and providing relief of the symptoms and complications of reflux while permitting normal swallowing in the absence of side effects such as bloating and the inability to vomit. According to the results of several recent publications, the modified Nissen fundoplication can be expected to produce these results in over 90% of patients for up to 10 years,[1] exceeding the results achieved with medical therapy.[2]

These excellent results, unfortunately, have not been uniformly experienced because persistent or recurrent symptoms occur in up to 23% of patients.[3] These treatment failures can be traced to problems related to patient selection and choice of operative procedure, as well as technical errors occurring in the course of the operation. These causes of failure can be prevented in most cases by strict adherence to well-documented criteria for patient selection and avoidance of undocumented modifications in technique.

Although the results of remedial operations for persistent or recurrent symptoms following failed antireflux procedures are less satisfying than the results following primary operations, careful evaluation and treatment can result in a satisfactory outcome. When the cause of failure is identified and addressed by appropriate surgical technique, 70% to 85% of patients can be expected to experience relief of their symptoms.

PREVENTION OF FAILURE OF PRIMARY ANTIREFLUX PROCEDURES
Errors in Patient Selection

The excellent results that have been achieved in several recent series demonstrate that when patients are appropriately selected, and procedures are properly performed, most failures can be prevented. The most important aspect of prevention is ensuring that the patient does, in fact, suffer from gastroesophageal reflux. To establish this, 24-hour ambulatory esophageal pH monitoring is essential, since symptoms have been shown to correlate poorly with the presence of reflux.[4] Likewise, reliance only on the presence of endoscopic evidence of esophageal injury will fail to recognize patients who may benefit from symptom control in the absence of complications. Endoscopic evaluation may also result in subjecting patients with primary esophageal motor disorders,[4] or drug-induced esophageal injury,[5] to procedures that are unnecessary.

To avoid these errors, thorough preoperative evaluation should be performed in all patients considered for antireflux surgery. Criteria for consideration of patients for fundoplication include the documentation of pathologic esophageal acid exposure on pH monitoring, demonstration of a mechanically defective lower esophageal sphincter (LES), and adequate propulsive motility in the esophageal body. Patients who have positive pH studies, but normal LES characteristics, should not undergo antireflux procedures. Rather, a search for other causes of increased esophageal acid exposure should be sought. The presence of delayed gastric emptying, gastric hypersecretion, poor esophageal clearance, or deficiency of saliva should be identified by appropriate testing.

Errors in Choice of Operative Procedure

Even when careful preoperative evaluation documents the presence of pathologic reflux, reflux symptoms may not be relieved, or symptoms of dysphagia may

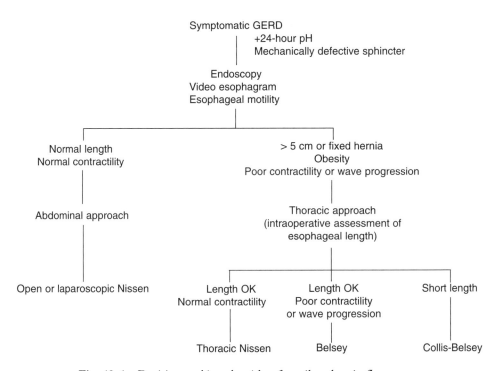

Fig. 13-1   Decision-making algorithm for tailored antireflux surgery.

emerge, if the proper procedure is not performed. In addition to avoiding an antireflux procedure in patients with primary gastric pathology, specific disorders of esophageal motility should be sought. This will avoid performing an obstructive fundoplication, such as a Nissen, in patients with poor motility, the cause of failure in 5% to 10% of patients[4,6] (Fig. 13-1).

Technical Errors

The final reason for persistent or recurrent symptoms following antireflux surgery is technical error. Technical errors include failure to recognize and treat appropriately patients with a shortened esophagus, failure to properly mobilize the esophagus and fundus adequately to avoid tension, and failure to adhere to the documented principles of constructing the fundoplication to avoid dysphagia[7] (Table 13-1).

Esophageal shortening, usually a manifestation of long-standing reflux disease and panmural fibrosis, has been shown to be a common cause of failure following fundoplication. Esophageal shortening may result in incorrect identification of the gastroesophageal junction, especially when excessive traction is made on the stomach. This results in the placement of the fundoplication around the proximal stomach rather than the gastroesophageal junction. This error is often referred to as a "slipped Nissen," but in reality is nearly always a misplaced wrap. Prevention of this problem requires identification of a shortened esophagus preoperatively. Endoscopic findings of a 5 cm or more hiatal hernia, or upper gastrointestinal evidence of a hernia that is not reducible, should alert the physician to the possibility of esophageal shortening. In these patients, a transthoracic approach should be used to allow complete mobilization of the thoracic esophagus. If the shortening is severe, a Collis gastroplasty can be added. Failure to identify the gastroesophageal junction at the time of repair can also result in a misplaced wrap. To avoid this problem, the esophageal fat pad is a useful landmark and should be mobilized com-

Table 13-1   Reasons for failure in 65 patients scheduled for remedial surgery for failed antireflux procedures (70 operations in 65 patients)*

Reasons for Failure	No. of Procedures (%)
Placement of wrap around stomach	22 (31)
Disrupted fundoplication	17 (24)
Herniation of repair into chest	12 (17)
Too long or too tight a wrap	5 (7)
Operative damage to lower esophagus	4 (6)
Primary motility disorder of the esophagus	5 (7)
Ineffective but intact repair	5 (7)
	70

*From Collard JM, Peters JH, Kauer WKH, DeMeester TR. Analysis of failed antireflex procedures and determinants of successful remedial operations (unpublished data).

pletely. Placement of the wrap between the right vagus nerve and the esophagus helps to ensure that the fundoplication is not placed too low.

Disruption of the wrap is the second most common reason for technical failure. Disruption can occur either as a result of excessive tension or because of postoperative gastric distention and breakdown of the repair. Complete mobilization of the gastric fundus by division of the short gastric vessels avoids the former; and the use of pledgets with a ∪ stitch[8] prevents the latter.

Herniation of the wrap into the chest is the primary cause of failure in 15% to 20% of patients with failed antireflux repairs. This too can be related to tension, but more commonly is due to inadequate closure of the hiatus. An intrathoracic fundoplication is a particularly dangerous situation. Catastrophic complications, such as ischemia and perforation, or massive hemorrhage can occur.[9] To avoid herniation of the wrap, the hiatus should be closed with five or six sutures placed behind the esophagus, spaced so that the surgeon's finger just fits into the hiatus alongside the esophagus.

Finally, two important aspects of construction of the fundoplication deserve emphasis. The first involves the length of the fundoplication, which should be no more than 1 to 2 cm. Longer wraps have been shown to be associated with a higher prevalence of dysphagia.[10] Short-term postoperative dysphagia can also be reduced by calibration of the lumen with a 60 F bougie dilator.

ASSESSMENT OF PATIENTS FOR REMEDIAL SURGERY

Patients who have recurrent or persistent symptoms following an antireflux procedure require a comprehensive symptom evaluation and correlation with anatomic and pathophysiologic derangement prior to consideration for remedial surgery.

Symptomatic and Functional Assessment

The most common symptoms are persistent or recurrent heartburn and regurgitation, dysphagia, and/or abdominal discomfort occurring during and after meals. The onset of dysphagia typically occurs soon after a failed antireflux repair and suggests a faulty construction of the fundoplication or the lack of appreciation of a preexisting stenosis or motor disorder of the esophageal body. In contrast, heartburn, which tends to occur later, is more likely to be due to subsequent breakdown of the repair leading to recurrent reflux.

In addition to a detailed symptomatic assessment, a thorough functional evaluation is essential to determine the cause of the recurrent or persistent symptoms and to outline the appropriate therapy. Patients who present with persistent or recurrent heartburn commonly have abnormal esophageal acid exposure on 24-hour ambulatory pH testing as well as mechanically defective sphincters, as is the situation in patients with untreated gastroesophageal reflux disease. Poor esophageal motility, incomplete relaxation of the LES, or intrathoracic herniation can all be demonstrated by motility testing in patients who experience dysphagia.

Anatomic Assessment

A barium contrast study and endoscopic examination are the principal techniques for anatomic assessment prior to remedial surgery. The barium study allows definition of the patient's anatomy and identifies strictures, wrap disruption, and paraesophageal herniation.[11] Particular importance is placed on the definition of a short esophagus and the irreducibility of a residual hiatal hernia into the abdomen. The endoscopic examination complements radiology, providing additional information regarding the state of the esophageal and gastric mucosa and allowing assessment of the integrity of the previous fundoplication.[12]

MANAGEMENT OF FAILED ANTIREFLUX SURGERY
Medical Therapy

Medical management of recurrent heartburn is unlikely to be successful in patients who have undergone previous antireflux surgery. However, in patients with severe esophagitis, an aggressive course of medical therapy is warranted even if surgery is planned. Such therapy may allow resolution of esophagitis. Strictures can be dilated during the course of medical therapy prior to surgery. Esophageal dysmotility may be related to esophagitis and may improve following treatment, provided no structural changes have taken place in the esophageal musculature.

Dysphagia is usually due to a mechanical outflow resistance or poor esophageal motility for which no medical treatment is available. Dilation has been tried in some patients who have excessively tight fundoplications but the results are in general discouraging.

Surgical Therapy

Careful assessment of the patient's symptoms and objective evaluation of esophageal function allow a specific plan of surgical therapy to be selected based on the underlying pathophysiology, together with the findings at reoperation.

Choice of Operation

The preferred surgical approach in patients with prior failed antireflux operations is a left thoracotomy. This incision allows simultaneous exposure of the upper abdomen and chest when the diaphragm is taken down at its periphery. The esophagus can be adequately mobilized through this incision and a gastroplasty can be added if necessary. The adhesions related to the previous operation are also easily managed through the exposure provided.

The choice of surgical procedure is tailored to the individual patient. Consideration should be given to the reasons for failure of the primary operation, esophageal length, and the peristaltic function of the esophagus. Existing gastric pathology and the presence of end-stage esophageal disease are also important factors to be considered in planning the procedure.

Patients who have a misplaced wrap ("slipped" Nissen) require a careful assessment of esophageal length. The causes of a misplaced Nissen include unrecognized esophageal shortening and incomplete dissection of the gastroesophageal junction. If the esophagus is found to be short after complete takedown of the old repair, a Collis-Belsey procedure is recommended. When the fundoplication was simply placed too low despite an adequate length of the esophagus, the choice of procedure depends on esophageal motility results. A transthoracic Nissen is performed when peristaltic function is normal. A Belsey fundoplication, which is inherently less obstructive, is performed in patients with poor esophageal motor function.

A similar approach is used in patients with disruption of a previous fundoplication, herniation of the wrap into the chest, and/or dysphagia due to an excessively long or tight fundoplication. In the presence of these technical errors, judgment as to the cause (esophageal shortening or failure to mobilize the fundus) usually outlines specific remedial measures. Again, complete mobilization is accomplished and a lengthening procedure is added as needed. When an esophageal motor disorder has been identified as the cause of dysphagia following a primary procedure, remedial procedures are designed to correct the underlying motility problem. A myotomy combined with a partial fundoplication is performed in patients with previously unrecognized achalasia or esophageal spasm. In most cases, however, the impaired motility consists of a nonspecific motor disorder with decreased amplitude of contractions and frequent incomplete peristaltic sequences. In these patients no specific therapy exists for the motor disorder and a Belsey fundoplication, which is less obstructive than a Nissen fundoplication, is the procedure of choice.

Esophageal resection should be considered whenever a patient has extensive fibrosis with refractory strictures. In these patients, and in those who have failed two or more prior procedures, results of remedial procedures are less satisfying. Resection should also be considered in patients who have recurrent or refractory symptoms in the presence of Barrett's-type intestinal metaplasia. Restoration of swallowing function and relief of symptoms are achieved in these patients with the additional benefit of eliminating the risk of carcinoma and the need for regular endoscopic surveillance. To provide long-term durable swallowing function, a colonic interposition is recommended.[13] The use of vagal sparing techniques[14] in particular has resulted in excellent function.

Other resectional procedures are occasionally applicable. Vagotomy and antrectomy with Roux-en-Y reconstruction has been advocated as an alternative in complicated situations.[15] This effectively eliminates both acid and alkaline reflux. Although postgastrectomy syndromes may prove troublesome in some patients, overall results have been satisfactory in properly selected patients, with symptomatic improvement in 85% at a median of 4½ years of follow-up.

Total gastrectomy may be advisable in patients who have gastric pathology as the primary cause of reflux, and when inadvertent vagotomy has occurred at the initial operation. This procedure reliably alleviates both acid and bile reflux and restores swallowing function.

RESULTS OF REMEDIAL PROCEDURES

Application of these principles to the patient with recurrent or persistent symptoms following an antireflux procedure results in 70% to 85% satisfactory long-

Table 13-2 Outcome in 65 patients after first remedial operations with respect to symptom and esophageal contractility*

Symptom	Type of Remedial Procedure	No. of Patients	Percent With Good Outcome†
Heartburn alone	Antireflux	19	95
Heartburn and dysphagia	Antireflux	16	81
Dysphagia alone	Antireflux	15	66
Any symptom with poor esophageal contractility	Antireflux	13	61
Any symptom with good esophageal contractility	Antireflux	40	92
Any symptom with poor esophageal contractility	Resection and interposition	6	83

*Modified from Collard JM, Peters JH, Kauer WKH, DeMeester TR. Analysis of failed antireflux procedures and determinants of successful remedial operations (unpublished data).
†Asymptomatic or minor symptoms not requiring treatment.

term results.[16] Although these results are slightly less successful than those seen following primary operations, they are nonetheless acceptable. Table 13-2 summarizes the results of a series of 65 patients undergoing remedial procedures at the University of Southern California.[7] The major determinant of outcome appeared to be the presence of a motility disorder. When present, only 61% had a satisfactory outcome following remedial surgery compared to 92% when esophageal motor function was normal. Resection may be a better option in patients who have abnormal motility because this procedure was associated with a good outcome in five of six patients.

CONCLUSION

Careful symptomatic evaluation, detailed esophageal function studies, and thorough anatomic assessment is necessary to determine the cause of failure in patients with failed antireflux surgery. A selective approach to reoperation is applied by tailoring the procedure performed to the errors that caused the primary failure. Adherence to the technical principles outlined minimizes the need for reoperation by avoiding preventable causes of failure.

Although the results of reoperation are in general not as good as those seen following primary antireflux procedures, they are still satisfactory considering the complicated nature of the abnormality. Resection may be the preferred option for patients who have dysphagia related to impaired esophageal motility.

REFERENCES

1. DeMeester TR, Bonavina L, Albertucci M. Nissen fundoplication for gastroesophageal reflux disease. Evaluation of primary repair in 100 consecutive patients. Ann Surg 204:2-9, 1986.

2. Spechler SJ, and the Department of Veterans Affairs Gastroesophageal Reflux Disease Study Group #277. Comparison of medical and surgical therapy for complicated gastroesophageal reflux disease in veterans. N Engl J Med 326:786-792, 1992.

3. Luostarinen ME, Isolauri JO, Koskinen MO, Laitinen JO, Matikeinen MJ, Lindholm TS. Refundoplication for recurrent gastroesophageal reflux. World J Surg 17:587-593, 1993.

4. Costantini M, Crookes PF, Bremner RM, Hoeft SF, Ehsan A, Peters JH, Bremner CG, DeMeester TR. The value of physiological assessment of foregut symptoms in a surgical practice. Surgery 114:780-787, 1993.

5. Bonavina L, DeMeester TR, McChesney L, Schwizer W, Albertucci M, Bailey RT. Drug induced esophageal strictures. Ann Surg 206:173, 1987.

6. DeMeester TR, Stein HJ. Surgical treatment of gastroesophageal reflux disease. In Castell DP, ed. The Esophagus. Boston: Little Brown, 1992, p 620.

7. Collard JM, Peters JH, Kauer WKH, DeMeester TR. Analysis of failed antireflux procedures and determinants of successful remedial operations (unpublished data).

8. DeMeester TR. Transthoracic antireflux procedures. In Nyhus LM, Baker RJ, eds. Mastery of Surgery. Boston: Little Brown, 1984, pp 381-392.

9. Richardson JD, Larson GM, Polk HC. Intrathoracic fundoplication for shortened esophagus: Treacherous solution to a challenging problem. Am J Surg 149:29, 1982.

10. DeMeester TR, Stein HJ. Minimizing the side effects of antireflux surgery. World J Surg 16:335-336, 1992.

11. Hatfield M, Shapir J. The radiologic manifestations of failed antireflux operations. AJR 144:1209, 1985.

12. O'Hanrahan T, Marples M, Bancewicz J. Recurrent reflux and wrap disruption after Nissen fundoplication: Detection, incidence, and timing. Br J Surg 150:248, 1985.

13. DeMeester TR, Johansson KE, Franze I. Indications, surgical technique, and long-term functional results of colonic interposition or bypass. Ann Surg 208:460-474, 1988.

14. Akiyama H, Tsurumaru M, Ono Y, et al. Esophagectomy without thoracotomy with vagal preservation. J Am Coll Surg 178:83-85, 1994.

15. Ellis FH, Gibb SP. Vagotomy, antrectomy, and Roux-en-Y diversion for complex reoperative gastroesophageal reflux disease. Ann Surg 220:536-543, 1994.

16. Little AG. Reoperation for failed repairs. In Pearson FG, ed. Esophageal Surgery. New York: Churchill Livingstone, 1995, pp 371-378.

14

Indication and Technique of Total Duodenal Diversion in Benign Esophageal Disease

Karl H. Fuchs, M.D. • *Johannes Heimbucher*, M.D.
Stephan M. Freys, M.D. • *Martin Fein*, M.D.

Duodenal diversion is most frequently used after total gastrectomy for reconstruction of the upper gastrointestinal tract.[1,2] Roux-en-Y reconstruction has been successfully used with an acceptable to excellent long-term quality of life in patients who have major foregut dysfunction.[3,4] The use of total duodenal diversion operation has, however, been very restricted in benign esophageal disease.[5]

The possible need for a duodenal diversion in gastroesophageal reflux disease (GERD) is limited to patients who have a combined foregut functional defect at the antroduodenal and gastroesophageal junctions.[6,7] There is increasing evidence that GERD can be caused or aggravated by a number of gastric functional disorders, such as abnormal gastric acidity,[8,9] delayed gastric emptying,[10] and pathologic duodenogastric reflux.[6,11] However, the role of duodenogastric reflux in GERD has been controversial.[12-15]

BACKGROUND OF ALKALINE REFLUX

Gastroesophageal reflux has been differentiated into acidic, mixed (acidic and alkaline), and alkaline reflux by use of pH measurements.[16] However, the actual pH value in the esophageal lumen does not distinguish the precise reflux components. Esophageal pH monitoring is an excellent method to provide information about acid reflux. However, the pH environment in the esophagus is influenced by saliva, possibly even bicarbonate secretion from the esophageal mucosa, and acid and alkaline fluids, which may reflux from the gastric lumen.[17,18] Intraesophageal pH monitoring is therefore an accurate method only if alkaline components play a minor role.

Duodenogastric reflux is a physiologic phenomenon.[14,19] Since it is difficult to accurately measure duodenogastric reflux, and since there is so far no "gold standard" investigation method, a precise and well-accepted borderline between normal and abnormal remains unknown, even though promising diagnostic tests are being evaluated.[20-24] Excessive or pathologic duodenogastric reflux has been implied in the development of gastritis, gastric ulcer disease, dyspepsia, and even carcinoma.[25-29] The effect of pathologic duodenogastric reflux and its toxic components on the esophageal mucosa have been demonstrated in patients and in the experimental model.[26-30] Recent studies also suggest that Barrett's epithelium is caused by combined acid and alkaline gastroesophageal reflux.[24,29,30]

Although many facts are known about the association of alkaline duodenogastric and gastroesophageal reflux, the therapeutic implications are controversial. Two main reasons seem to be responsible for this situation.

First, the diagnosis of pathologic duodenogastric reflux, that is, the accurate assessment of this abnormal condition, is very difficult to establish. The detection of alkaline reflux and/or the detection of its different components have been difficult and unreliable.[15,22,23] The presence of bile salts as measured in the aspirated gastric and esophageal contents has been reported in many patients with esophagitis.[20,21] In contrast, some studies have not confirmed an increase in duodenal contents in the esophagus.[14] Three main investigative methods are currently used to detect alkaline duodenal components in the esophageal lumen: (1) the aspiration method[31]; (2) 24-hour combined esophageal and gastric pH monitoring[11]; and, more recently, (3) fiberoptic sensor 24-hour monitoring of bile for directly measuring bilirubin.[23]

Second, the most successful medical treatment of gastroesophageal reflux is to reduce acid in the esophageal lumen, and not the neutralization of toxic alkaline components such as bile and pancreatic enzymes.[32,33] As a consequence, clinicians have expressed doubts about the importance of alkaline reflux. The majority of reflux patients can be successfully treated with proton pump inhibitors and even H_2 receptor blockers. Antisecretory drugs heal esophagitis and diminish symptoms in up to 95% of patients. However, these drugs are markedly less successful in patients with severe complications, such as confluent esophagitis, stenoses, ulcers, and detectable Barrett's epithelium.[34] A reasonable explanation for the limitations in medical therapy in these patients is the increasing evidence that duodenogastroesophageal reflux also plays an important role in the pathogenesis of the disease.[35]

INDICATION FOR DUODENAL DIVERSION PROCEDURES IN GASTROESOPHAGEAL REFLUX DISEASE

Pathologic duodenogastric reflux can be detected in 10% to 30% of all reflux patients.[8,35] There is no place for a duodenal diversion in patients with primary reflux disease caused by an incompetent lower esophageal sphincter. Even if pathologic duodenogastroesophageal reflux has been documented in the preoperative investigations, caution should be exercised before a total duodenal diversion procedure is added to the fundoplication. Surgical augmentation of the lower esophageal sphincter to prevent possible acid and alkaline reflux into the esophagus has been reported to be successful in 85% of patients. This applies also to Barrett's patients in whom "alkaline" reflux can be detected in 60% of patients tested.[7] Since the success rate of a Nissen fundoplication can be as high as 90% to 95% in primary reflux patients with an isolated sphincter defect, one can speculate that the necessity for a combined total duodenal diversion procedure together with a fundoplication is likely to be very unusual.[6,7]

Patients with suspected duodenogastroesophageal reflux must be studied thoroughly using all current diagnostic measures to determine the probability of the pathophysiologic importance of such a finding. Indications for a duodenal diversion operation should be based on a spectrum of investigative results, including upper gastrointestinal endoscopy to detect ulcers, scars, strictures, or duodenal bulb deformities; esophageal manometry to detect esophageal peristaltic disorders and lower esophageal sphincter incompetency; antroduodenal manometry to verify gastric and antroduodenal motility disorders; 24-hour esophageal and gastric pH monitoring to confirm acid and alkaline reflux; fiberoptic 24-hour bile monitoring of the esophagus and stomach; gastric-emptying scintigraphy for evidence of delayed gastric emptying; and a barium study to detect gastric wall abnormalities. If excessive alkaline reflux into the esophageal lumen is identified, the patient should be clearly informed that the planned antireflux operation, usually a Nissen fundoplication, may possibly be only the first step of the procedures that are necessary to bring constant relief. A preoperative therapeutic trial of medical therapy to neutralize or prevent alkaline-refluxed components often acts as a diagnostic guide in the individual patient.

A duodenal diversion operation is indicated only in symptomatic patients who have had a history of continued reflux disease after medical therapy and have clearly documented duodenogastric reflux. Depending on the individual patient, a Roux-en-Y suprapapillary duodenojejunostomy preserving the stomach and pylorus or a distal gastric resection and Roux-en-Y reconstruction are the procedures employed.[36-38] The decision to select one or the other procedure must be based on accompanying gastric pathology and gastric function. If there is evidence for abnormal gastric motility with excessively delayed emptying and altered gastric morphology or gastric outlet obstruction, a distal gastric resection is advisable. On the other hand, if an antroduodenal motility disorder causing excessive duodenogastric reflux is detected, and if gastric and duodenal function and morphology are normal, it is reasonable to perform the stomach-preserving duodenal switch operation.

The most important indication for a total duodenal diversion procedure is a failed previous antireflux procedure and evidence of alkaline reflux into the esophageal lumen causing complications. In such circumstances a Roux-en-Y suprapapillary duodenojejunostomy to divert the alkaline juice is indicated, provided that no other gastric problems are detected.

If previous gastric surgery has been performed, a distal gastric resection or even completion total gastrectomy must be considered. Altered gastric function due to previous surgery, scarring, and adhesions around the duodenal bulb and the head of the pancreas will make a dissection for a suprapapillary duodenojejunostomy impractical.

Excessive enterogastric reflux following a Billroth II gastrojejunostomy will require disconnection of the afferent jejunal or duodenal loop and a Roux-en-Y reconstruction with vagotomy.

Gastroesophageal reflux associated with ineffective esophageal body motility is best treated surgically by a partial fundoplication, which is less obstructive. Such a partial repair does not completely control alkaline reflux and if persistent symptoms continue or complications develop, a duodenal diversion should be considered.

In summary, the indication for a total duodenal diversion procedure must be limited to a very select group of patients. These patients must be studied very carefully to document excessive alkaline reflux. All diagnostic possibilities and the experience of the laboratory and surgical center must be used before a patient is selected to have duodenal diversion surgery.

TECHNIQUE OF TOTAL DUODENAL DIVERSION COMBINED WITH ANTIREFLUX PROCEDURES
Roux-en-Y Suprapapillary Duodenojejunostomy (Duodenal Switch Operation) and Fundoplication

The two procedures have been described previously.[6,36] When a combined procedure is planned, it is probably advisable to perform the Nissen fundoplication first to reduce the necessary manipulation of the duodenojejunostomy. In many of these patients, a revision fundoplication might be necessary and any surgical procedure at the gastroesophageal junction should be performed without the risk of disruption of the duodenal switch operation. The combination of these operations at one time should be an exception. Often the patient in question has a mechanically intact fundoplication at the gastroesophageal junction, but has persistent alkaline reflux problems.

Our preference is to perform the biliary diversion procedure through a bilateral subcostal upper abdominal incision, but other authors prefer an upper midline incision. When the Roux-en-Y suprapapillary duodenojejunostomy is begun, the duodenum is mobilized by a Kocher maneuver to feel the head of the pancreas and especially the position of the papilla of Vater as accurately as possible. Care must be taken to dissect an area around the duodenum well above the papilla and without devascularizing the proximal duodenum. Using the thumb and index finger around the duodenum, it is usually possible to feel the closest approximation at a point along the medial duodenal border just proximal to the papilla at approximately 3 to 7 cm distal to the pylorus, depending on the anatomic situation of the patient. At this point the duodenum is dissected free of the head of the pancreas by carefully dividing the small vessels. Precautions must also be taken to avoid damage to the intrapancreatic common bile duct.

When the channel between pancreatic head and duodenum is completed, the duodenum can easily be divided and closed with a linear stapling device. Since the dissection is carried down to the most distal point just proximal of the papilla, it is not advisable to oversew the stapling suture to avoid obstruction of the common bile duct.

The first or second jejunal loop, depending on the vascular status of the mesentery, is pulled supracolically into the area of the duodenal bulb through an opening in the transverse mesocolon, and to the right of the midcolic vessels (Fig. 14-1). A dissection point in the jejunal loop is identified to prepare a limb that is long

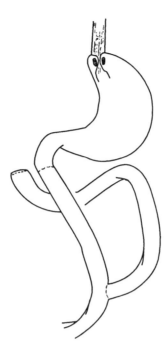

Fig. 14-1 Concept of total duodenal diversion by Roux-en-Y suprapapillary duodenojejunostomy, the duodenal switch operation. The operation can be combined with the classic antireflux procedures at the gastroesophageal junction.

enough to complete the Roux-en-Y jejunojejunostomy without tension. The distal jejunal loop is then sutured to the proximal duodenal stump in an end-to-end anastomosis. The proximal jejunal limb is anastomosed end-to-side to the distal jejunal limb 40 to 50 cm distal to the duodenojejunal anastomosis. The opening in the mesocolon is closed.

Distal Gastric Resection and Roux-en-Y Reconstruction and Antireflux Procedures

This procedure is indicated in symptomatic patients with GERD following previous operations of the stomach or antroduodenal area or GERD associated with gastroduodenal ulcer disease. These patients have usually had antireflux procedures combined with vagotomy, pyloroplasty, or antrectomy to correct a functional defect or excise the ulcer-bearing segment of the stomach. Previous surgery may even have aggravated existing alkaline reflux. The optimal procedure in these patients is dependent on what can be done at the gastroesophageal junction. It is often impossible to use the fundus to perform a regular Nissen fundoplication because of the limited size of the gastric stump. A Hill posterior gastropexy operation or a partial fundoplication can be used to improve the antireflux barrier at the gastroesophageal junction.[39-41]

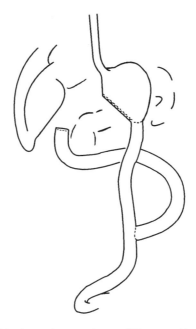

Fig. 14-2   Distal gastric resection and Roux-en-Y reconstruction.

If the fundoplication is intact, the distal part of the stomach is resected, using a linear stapling device. The first or second jejunal loop is mobilized and the distal jejunal limb is brought through an opening in the transverse mesocolon. We perform a gastrojejunostomy (Fig. 14-2) with one row of seromuscular 4-0 absorbable suture material. As an alternative, a circular stapling device with a 28 mm cartridge or a biofragmentable ring anastomotic device, again with 28 mm diameter, can be used. The opening in the mesentery approximated to the jejunum and the Roux-en-Y jejunojejunostomy is performed end-to-side using a running suture of 4-0 absorbable material or a biofragmentable ring anastomosis.

In the preoperative diagnostic workup, it is important to analyze the acid output to ensure sufficient acid suppression to prevent peptic jejunal ulceration in the efferent limb. In their first series of suprapapillary duodenojejunostomies De-Meester et al.[36] only reported on one patient who developed a jejunal ulcer after the duodenal switch operation. This patient had a preoperative hyperacidity and subsequently was successfully treated with a highly selective vagotomy. Truncal vagotomy is always necessary when antrectomy or revision gastrectomy is reconstructed with a Roux-en-Y procedure.[35]

CONCLUSION

There is still uncertainty about the precise pathophysiologic role that toxic alkaline reflux components play in the cause of esophagitis, especially esophageal carcinoma.[42] This uncertainty is related to a lack of the precise assessment of alkaline reflux. Promising technical developments and studies in the past 3 years have led to current optimism that these diagnostic problems could be solved within the next 5 years.[43] The routine use of duodenal diversion operations can only be based on precise diagnostic data and proof of pathologic duodenogastric reflux.

REFERENCES

1. Herfarth CH, Schlag P, Buhl K. Surgical procedures for gastric substitution. World J Surg 11:689-698, 1987.
2. Thiede A, Fuchs KH, Hamelmann H. Pouch and Roux-en-Y reconstruction after gastrectomy: Systematic use of staplers in stomach replacement. Arch Surg 122:837-842, 1987.
3. Troidl H, Kusche J, Vestweber JH, et al. Pouch versus oesophagojejunostomy after total gastrectomy: A randomized clinical trial. World J Surg 11:699-712, 1987.
4. Roder JD, Heschbach P, Henrich G, et al. Lebensqualität nach totaler Gastrektomie wegen Magenkarzinoms. Dtsch Med Wochenschr 117:241-247, 1992.
5. Hinder RA, Bremner CG. The uses and consequences of the Roux-en-Y operation. Surg Annu 19:151-174, 1987.
6. DeMeester TR. Definition, detection and pathophysiology of gastroesophageal reflux disease. In DeMeester TR, Matthews HR, eds. International Trends in General Thoracic Surgery. Benign Esophageal Disease, vol. 3. St. Louis: CV Mosby, 1987, pp 99-127.
7. DeMeester TR, Attwood SEA, Smyrk TC, et al. Surgical therapy in Barrett's esophagus. Ann Surg 212:528-542, 1990.
8. Fuchs KH, Eypasch EP, DeMeester TR, et al. Differentiation of esophagitis grade IV—What is the background? [abstract]. Surg Endosc 2:113, 1988.
9. Barlow AP, DeMeester TR, Boll CS, et al. The significance of the gastric secretory state in gastroesophageal reflux disease. Arch Surg 124:937-940, 1989.
10. Schwizer W, Hinder RA, DeMeester TR. Does delayed gastric emptying contribute to gastroesophageal reflux disease? Am J Surg 157:74-81, 1989.
11. Fuchs KH, DeMeester TR, Albertucci M, et al. Quantification of the duodenogastric reflux in gastroesophageal reflux disease. In Siewart JR, Holscher AH, eds. Diseases of the Esophagus. New York: Springer-Verlag, 1987, pp 831-835.
12. Pellegrini CA, DeMeester TR, Wernly JA, et al. Alkaline gastro-esophageal reflux. Am J Surg 135:177-184, 1978.
13. Gowen GW. Spontaneous enterogastric reflux gastritis and esophagitis. Ann Surg 201:170-175, 1985.
14. Blum AL, Heading R, Müller-Lissner S, et al. Is duodenogastric reflux clinically relevant? Gastroenterol Int 2:1-8, 1989.
15. Bremner CG, Mason RJ. "Bile" in the oesophagus. Br J Surg 80:1374-1376, 1993.
16. Mattioli S, Pilotti V, Felice V, et al. Ambulatory 24-hr pH monitoring of the esophagus, fundus, and antrum. Dig Dis Sci 35:929-938, 1990.
17. Meyers RL, Orlando RC. Bicarbonate secretion by human esophagus. Gastroenterology 102:A126, 1992.
18. Singh S, Bradley LA, Richter JE. Determinants of oesophageal "alkaline" pH environment in controls and patients with gastro-oesophageal reflux disease. Gut 34:309-316, 1993.
19. Müller-Lissner SA, Fimmel CJ, Sonnenberg A, et al. Novel approach to quantify duodenogastric reflux in healthy volunteers and in patients with type I gastric ulcer. Gut 24:510-518, 1983.
20. Gillison EW, Capper WM, Airth GR, et al. Hiatus hernia and heartburn. Gut 10:609-613, 1969.
21. Gotley DC, Morgan AP, Cooper MJ. Bile acid concentration in the refluxate of patients with reflux oesophagitis. Br J Surg 75:587-590, 1988.
22. Fuchs KH, DeMeester TR, Hinder RA, et al. Computerized identification of pathological duodenogastric reflux using 24-hour gastric pH monitoring. Ann Surg 213:13-20, 1991.

23. Bechi P, Pucciani F, Baldini F, et al. Long-term ambulatory enterogastric reflux monitoring—Validation of a new fiberoptic technique. Dig Dis Sci 38:1297-1306, 1993.
24. Stein HJ, Barlow AP, DeMeester TR, et al. Complications in gastroesophageal reflux disease. Role of the lower esophageal sphincter, duodenogastric reflux and esophageal acid and alkaline exposure. Ann Surg 216:35-43, 1992.
25. Du Plessis DH. Pathogenesis of gastric ulceration. Lancet 1:974-978, 1965.
26. Rhodes J, Barnardo DE, Philips SF, et al. Increased reflux of bile into the stomach in patients with gastric ulcer. Gastroenterology 57:241-252, 1969.
27. Ritchie WP Jr. Alkaline reflux gastritis: Late results on a controlled trial of diagnosis and treatment. Ann Surg 203:537-544, 1986.
28. Bost R, Hostein J, Valenti M, et al. Is there an abnormal lasting duodenogastric reflux in nonulcer dyspepsia? Dig Dis Sci 35:193-199, 1990.
29. Yasui A, Hoeft SF, DeMeester TR, et al. An alkaline stomach is common to Barrett's esophagus and gastric carcinoma. Gastroenterology 102:A411, 1992.
30. Attwood SEA, Barlow AP, Norris TL, et al. Barrett's oesophagus: Effect of antireflux surgery on symptom control and development of complications. Br J Surg 79:1060, 1992.
31. Stein HJ, Feussner H, Kauer W, et al. Alkaline gastroesophageal reflux: Assessment by ambulatory esophageal aspiration and pH monitoring. Am J Surg 167:163-168, 1994.
32. Klinkenberg-Knol EC, Meuwissen SGM. Treatment of reflux oesophagitis resistant to H_2-receptor antagonists. Digestion 44:47, 1989.
33. Koop H, Arnold R. Long-term maintenance treatment of reflux esophagitis with omeprazole. Prospective study with H_2-blocker-resistant esophagitis. Dig Dis Sci 36:552, 1991.
34. Bell NIV, Hunt RH. Role of gastric acid suppression in the treatment of gastro-oesophageal reflux disease. Gut 33:118-124, 1992.
35. Peters JH, Kauer WKH, DeMeester TR. Alkaline gastroesophageal reflux. Therapeutic options for patients with alkaline gastro-esophageal reflux. Dis Esoph 7:93-98, 1994.
36. DeMeester TR, Fuchs KH, Ball CS, et al. Experimental and clinical results with proximal end-to-end duodenojejunostomy for pathologic duodenogastric reflux. Ann Surg 206:414-426, 1987.
37. Tanner NC, Westerholm P. Partial gastrectomy in the treatment of esophageal stricture after hiatal hernia. Am J Surg 115:449-453, 1968.
38. Hinder RA, Esser J, DeMeester TR. Management of gastric emptying disorders following the Roux-en-Y procedure. Surgery 104:765-772, 1988.
39. Hill LD. Intraoperative measurement of lower esophageal sphincter pressure. J Thorac Cardiovasc Surg 75:378-382, 1978.
40. DeMeester TR, Fuchs KH. Comparison of operations for uncomplicated reflux disease. In Jamieson GG, ed. Surgery of the Oesophagus. New York: Churchill Livingstone, 1988, pp 299-308.
41. Fuchs KH. Operative procedures in antireflux surgery. Endosc Surg 1:65-71, 1993.
42. Attwood SEA. Alkaline gastro-esophageal reflux and esophageal carcinoma: Experimental evidence and clinical implications. Dis Esoph 7:87-92, 1994.
43. Stein HJ, Feussner H. Diagnostic approach to "alkaline" gastro-esophageal reflux. Dis Esoph 7:80-86, 1994.

15

Esophageal Replacement for Benign Disease

Thomas J. Watson, M.D. • *Werner K.H. Kauer, M.D.*
Tom R. DeMeester, M.D.

End-stage esophageal disease has a profound effect on the patient's nutrition and ability to lead a normal and fulfilled life. Persons who suffer from the effects of severe esophageal disorders or previously failed esophageal surgery are often prescribed a myriad of ineffective medications in the hope of alleviating distressing symptomatology. These desperate and unfortunate patients are often referred from one physician to the next in search of a cure. The only therapeutic hope, however, for these individuals is surgical intervention. Because previous surgery has often contributed to the problem, both patient and physician are reluctant to accept further complex surgical therapy that may have a touted high mortality and questionable outcome. In our experience, esophageal replacement for benign disease can be safely performed, with minimal morbidity and mortality and with excellent long-term functional results. This chapter examines the characteristics of the patient population considered for esophagectomy, the surgical principles requisite to the successful reconstruction of the foregut, as well as the safety and outcome of the various reconstructive alternatives.

PATIENT CHARACTERISTICS

Our cumulative experience with esophageal replacement for benign disease has recently been reviewed. In total, 87 patients with end-stage benign esophageal disease underwent surgical reconstruction. There were 51 males and 36 females ranging in age from 6 to 79 years (median, 44 years). Seventy-five patients (86%) had at least one previous esophageal operation with a median of two and a maximum of 12. The most common initial procedure was an ineffective antireflux operation. In our experience, once a person has undergone three unsuccessful antireflux repairs, a fourth is destined to failure and an esophagectomy is invariably indicated.

In 90% of the patients, the major factor driving surgery was persistent dysphagia, 56% of whom had already been treated with one or more dilations. Other causes for referral were aspiration, fistula, or perforation. Patients presented with a variety of foregut symptoms (Table 15-1). The primary abnormality responsible for these symptoms was a severe end-stage motility disorder in 26 patients, an undilat-

Table 15-1 Symptoms of end-stage esophageal disease in 87 patients

Symptom	%
Dysphagia	90
Regurgitation	57
Heartburn	52
Weight loss	32
Chest pain	25
Epigastric pain	22
Vomiting	20
Coughing	18
Nausea	18
Choking	9
Voice change	7
Diarrhea	3
Odynophagia	2
Anorexia	1
Bloating	1

able peptic or drug-induced stricture in 25 patients, deterioration from long-term gastroesophageal reflux disease (GERD) in 11 patients, traumatic or spontaneous perforation in 11 patients, corrosive injury in eight patients, congenital abnormality in five patients, and an aortoesophagocutaneous fistula following correction of aortic coarctation in one patient.

Some clinical judgment may be required in deciding which patients should undergo esophagectomy. The patient's symptomatology must be sufficiently severe to warrant a major resection and reconstruction in the face of a benign disease. Most patients, however, have exhausted attempts at "conservative" management by nonsurgeons at the time of referral to a surgical specialist. The mere fact that these patients finally present to a surgeon often reflects the magnitude of the underlying disease process and the desire to seek a cure, even if a major operation is the only solution.

PREOPERATIVE EVALUATION

The functional status of the foregut is routinely evaluated prior to elective reconstruction using video upper gastrointestinal barium contrast studies, esophagogastroduodenoscopy, and stationary esophageal motility, 24-hour esophageal, and/or gastric pH monitoring. Ambulatory esophageal motility studies are obtained when further detailed information regarding esophageal body function is essential to making a therapeutic decision. Gastric emptying is evaluated when symptoms or results of function studies suggest gastroparesis.

The patient's cardiopulmonary reserve must be assessed prior to performing an extensive esophageal resection and reconstruction. Although the importance of a thorough history and complete physical examination cannot be overemphasized, neither is sufficient to detect subtle deficiencies in cardiopulmonary function that might prove significant in the face of substantial perioperative stress. Consequently, a more objective evaluation of the heart and lungs is imperative in all patients over 50 years of age, as well as in any person with symptoms suggestive of underlying cardiopulmonary disease. Pulmonary function testing is routinely performed in all such patients and a forced expiratory volume of less than 1.25 L is considered a relative contraindication to surgery. Likewise, the heart is routinely evaluated using stress echocardiography or multigated nuclear (MUGA) scanning. A resting cardiac ejection fraction of 0.40 that drops further on exercise is considered an unfavorable prognostic indicator.

Patients considered for colonic interposition as the method of esophageal replacement undergo colonoscopy to evaluate the status of the colonic mucosa. The presence of mild diverticular disease does not preclude the use of the colon, although frank diverticulitis or extensive diverticulosis, especially if associated with inflammatory fibrosis, is a contraindication to colonic interposition. In addition, the presence of a few colonic polyps, whether hyperplastic or adenomatous, that can be removed before surgery does not preclude the use of colon, but the presence of extensive polyposis or malignancy is a contraindication.

Because adequate arterial anatomy of the colon is essential to a successful colon interposition, preoperative mesenteric arteriography is mandatory in patients considered potential candidates for such a procedure. The study should include selective injections of the celiac axis and the superior and inferior mesenteric arteries, paying particular attention to anatomic aberrancies. The most important is the status of the inferior mesenteric artery, especially in older patients with atherosclerosis. Significant atherosclerotic changes involving the origin and initial portion of this vessel are contraindications to the use of the left colon as an esophageal substitute and alternative sources should be sought. A segment of right colon based on the middle colic vessels can often be used instead of the standard left colonic segment based on the inferior mesenteric artery and vein. The marginal artery in the region of the splenic flexure is also carefully assessed because this important arcade is absent or incomplete in 5% of patients. Similarly, the anatomy of the middle colic vessels, as well as their anastomotic arcades with the right colic vasculature, must be defined because there is much variability.

CHOICE OF ESOPHAGEAL SUBSTITUTE
Stomach Versus Colon

Most surgeons use the stomach for esophageal reconstruction if it is intact. We prefer to use the colon, if it is available, particularly if the replacement must last a decade or longer. To date, we have performed 71 colon interpositions and only four gastric pull-ups as reconstructions for benign esophageal disease (Figs. 15-1 and 15-2). The techniques used have been reported previously.[1,2]

A gastric advancement is without doubt the best esophageal replacement when esophagectomy is performed for palliation of cancer and long-term survival is unlikely. The extent of operative dissection and the resultant physiologic insult are

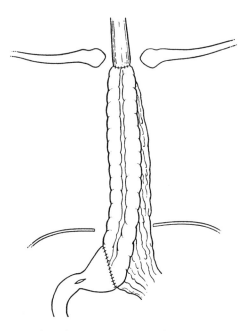

Fig. 15-1 Schematic drawing of a colon interposition. The proximal gastric resection depicted was added later in the series.

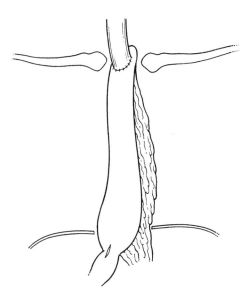

Fig. 15-2 Schematic drawing of a gastric pull-up with a cervical esophagogastrostomy. In most situations this was performed through the transhiatal approach.

less when preparing the stomach for advancement compared to the colon. The in-hospital recovery and time to return of unrestricted alimentation are also probably shorter in patients undergoing the gastric pull-up procedure.

Controversy exists, however, as to whether colon or stomach is a better long-term substitute for the esophagus in patients with benign disease. In our opinion, an intrathoracic stomach is a poor long-term esophageal substitute. Although technically easier to perform, the gastric advancement is frequently associated with symptoms related to duodenogastric reflux and rapid gastric emptying in the upright position.[3] Most patients experience symptoms during or shortly after eating. The most common of these symptoms are a postprandial pressure sensation and early satiety, which is probably related to the loss of the gastric reservoir.

Our experience indicates that these symptoms are less common when the colon is used, probably because the distal third of the stomach remains in its normal position within the abdomen, resulting in slower gastric emptying, and the interposed colon functions as an additional reservoir. Following a gastric advancement, the pylorus lies at the level of the esophageal hiatus and a distinct intraluminal pressure gradient develops between the intra-abdominal duodenum and the intrathoracic stomach. Unless the pyloric valve is extremely efficient, the pressure differential encourages reflux of duodenal contents into the stomach. The addition of a pyloroplasty may intensify the problem. Duodenogastric reflux is less likely to occur following colonic interposition because the pylorus and duodenum are retained within their natural positions and there is sufficient intra-abdominal colon compressed by the positive intra-abdominal pressure to prevent reflux.

Dysphagia requiring dilation is more frequent when the stomach is used as the esophageal replacement. In a study by Orringer and Stirling[4] of 87 patients who underwent esophageal replacement using the stomach for benign disease, 54 patients (67%) required immediate postoperative dilation and 13 patients (15%) had persistent dysphagia requiring home dilation. In comparison, only four of 71 patients (6%) with a colon interposition required immediate dilation and none had persistent dysphagia requiring home dilation. Although a minority of patients with a colon interposition may experience a sensation of slow transit, this is caused by eating at a speed exceeding the colon's ability to transport the swallowed bolus rather than an obstruction to the passage of a bolus as experienced by patients with a gastric pull-up.

The late development of proximal esophagitis, stenosis, or Barrett's esophagus is more common with an esophagogastric anastomosis made within the chest.[5] For this reason alone an intrathoracic esophagogastrostomy should be abandoned. We never perform an Ivor Lewis–type esophagectomy with an intrathoracic esophagogastrostomy. Although there is general acceptance of the concept that an esophagogastric anastomosis in the neck results in less postoperative esophagitis and stricture formation than one performed within the chest, reflux esophagitis following a cervical anastomosis does occur. Patients undergoing a cervical esophagogastrostomy for benign disease can develop problems associated with the anastomosis in the fourth or fifth postoperative year that may be severe enough to require anastomotic revision.

Such stricturing is uncommon in patients who have had a colon interposition for esophageal replacement. The interposed colon functions to protect the remaining esophagus from refluxed gastric juice. This may be related to mucous production and to the fact that its intra-abdominal segment remains collapsed because of positive intra-abdominal pressures. Long-term studies have shown that the colon appears to undergo little if any histologic change when used as an esophageal substitute.[6] Consequently, in patients with benign disease a colon interposition is preferred to obviate the late problems associated with esophagogastrostomy.

Vagal-Sparing Esophagectomy

The most compelling reason for not using the stomach to reestablish gastrointestinal continuity is that a vagotomy must be performed with all its inherent complications.[7] Many of the annoyances that occur after esophageal replacement are because of the concomitant vagotomy and the loss of parasympathetic modulation of foregut function. If the vagus nerves are intact, they should be preserved by performing a vagal-sparing esophagectomy[8] (Fig. 15-3). This is accomplished by dividing the esophagus in the neck and at the gastroesophageal junction in the abdomen, sparing the vagal nerves. The isolated esophagus is removed by passing a vein stripper up through the esophagus via a small incision in the cardia, securing it to the distal portion of the divided cervical esophagus, and invaginating the esophagus as it is pulled through the esophageal hiatus of the diaphragm. The va-

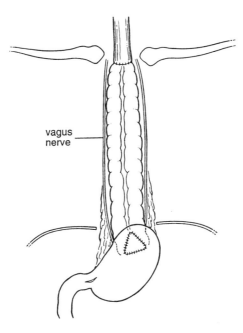

vagus
nerve

Fig. 15-3 Schematic drawing of a vagal-sparing esophagectomy with colon interposition. This reconstruction appears to give the best postoperative function.

gal nerves are sheared off as the muscular wall turns in during the invagination process. The remaining posterior mediastinal tunnel is progressively dilated with a 90 ml Foley catheter to create an adequate passageway for the colon interposition graft. Using this technique, the colon is anastomosed to a fully innervated stomach. Of course, this procedure is only applicable when the vagi have not been previously compromised and the patient does not otherwise suffer from gastroparesis. Based on early results of the vagal-sparing esophagectomy and colon interposition in several patients, and its theoretical advantages, we believe it is the operation of choice for esophageal reconstruction when it can be technically accomplished, when the patient is physiologically fit, and when long-term esophageal function is sought.

Colon Interposition to the Denervated Stomach

A more common situation arises when the vagi have been divided and part of the stomach has been resected by prior surgery. A colon interposition anastomosed to such a stomach is destined to encounter regurgitation of gastric contents. Because many of the problems ascribed to colon interposition are merely a result of poor gastric emptying, a two thirds proximal gastrectomy is routinely performed whenever a colon is interposed to a denervated stomach. The remaining distal third of the stomach is anastomosed end-to-end to the colon graft. This technique results in a better functional result because the colonic interposition serves as a contracting reservoir for the retained antrum, which continues its own innate contractions at three cycles per minute, thereby maintaining its pump function. Postoperative gastroparesis and delayed gastric emptying, which occurs when more of the stomach is retained, are avoided. This adverse effect of delayed gastric emptying was demonstrated late in our experience and, as a consequence, a proximal gastrectomy has been combined with a colon interposition only in our most recent patients. Nonetheless, the outcome in these patients is impressive compared to the previous group in whom the stomach was left intact.

Choice of Colonic Segment

There is some controversy regarding the preferred colonic segment to be used for interposition. The appropriate choice depends on the reliability of the respective vascular pedicles, both arterial and venous, as well as whether the colon graft will be placed in an isoperistaltic or antiperistaltic orientation. In our opinion, the left colon based on the ascending branch of the left colic artery and the inferior mesenteric vein is the segment of choice. The concept of using long segments of colon to replace or bypass the esophagus was introduced independently by Kelling[9] and Vulliet[10] in 1911. Kelling described an isoperistaltic left colon transplant and Vulliet described an antiperistaltic graft using the transverse colon. Vulliet stated that his procedure was technically easier than the isoperistaltic alternatives and that the functional result was the same because the colon does not normally exhibit peristalsis. Since that time, studies have demonstrated that the colon is not simply an inert tube. It is active in peristalsis, especially when challenged by a number of stimuli, with a frequency that increases the longer it is in place. In fact, in patients with a long-standing antiperistaltic colon interposition, peristaltic movement of a barium bolus has been shown to proceed against gravity, toward the pharynx, resulting in choking and chronic aspiration. Consequently, an isoperistaltic-interposed colon should always be used. Although we prefer to use the left colon segment, the right colon, placed isoperistaltically and based on the middle colic vessels, may also be suitable if the left colon is unavailable or its vasculature is compromised.

Jejunal Interposition and Free Graft

The use of jejunum has been advocated as the esophageal substitute of choice. In our experience, the ability to ingest has been better with a colon compared with a jejunal graft and, consequently, only eight jejunal interpositions have been performed to date. Based on a postoperative questionnaire, patients with colon interpositions were able to eat more and were more likely to experience normal transit and less early satiety than those with jejunal interpositions (Table 15-2). These differences probably relate to the greater reservoir capacity of the colon consistent with its native function. The greater motility in the jejunal graft does little to improve transit and is more likely to cause nausea and bloating. Furthermore, the loss of a segment of colon does not result in more frequent stools.

An additional problem with jejunal interpositions is that they only reach proximally to approximately the sternal angle of Louis. Consequently, a substantial length of functional proximal esophagus must be retained and the anastomosis must be performed in an intrathoracic location. Satisfactory long-term functional results have not been obtained from jejunal interpositions placed within the posterior mediastinum and this route is not advocated. Substernal jejunal interpositions, on the other hand, function better but generally necessitate a median sternotomy. The additional exposure is requisite to performing the esophagojejunal anastomosis. If there is a choice, we again prefer to use the colon rather than jejunum for esophageal replacement.

Circumstances may arise when the colon and stomach are unavailable or unsuitable as an esophageal substitute and insufficient proximal esophagus remains to perform a jejunal interposition. A jejunal free graft remains the procedure of choice in such dire circumstances. Although our use of the free graft in reconstructions for benign esophageal disease has been limited, the accumulated experience after

Table 15-2 Comparison between types of interposition and ability to ingest

Assessment	Jejunum % (n = 6)	Colon % (n = 28)
Able to take three meals/day	67	89
Able to eat steak dinner	33	54
Normal transit	50	79
Free of satiety	17	46

esophagectomy for malignancies involving the upper aerodigestive tract indicates that it is the best of the remaining alternatives. The added complexity of the operation, including the need for microvascular anastomoses, makes it difficult to recommend jejunal free grafting when another organ is available for transposition or interposition.

Choice of Transthoracic Route

When colon or stomach is used as the esophageal substitute, the posterior mediastinal route is preferred instead of a substernal tunnel for transporting the organ to the neck. This route allows better drainage from the remaining cervical esophagus into the esophageal replacement and minimizes the amount of operative dissection. At times the posterior mediastinum is unavailable secondary to scarring from previous surgery; then the substernal route is mandated. If this latter route is chosen, a tunnel can usually be created safely using blunt dissection provided that there has not been previous scarring in the anterior mediastinum. If such scarring is present, a median sternotomy may be essential. The left half of the manubrium, the medial end of the first rib, and the sternal head of the left clavicle are routinely resected to enlarge the thoracic inlet. Care must be taken not to enter the pleura or destroy the internal mammary artery or vein, which may be needed as vascular pedicles for subsequent "supercharging" of a colon interposition, or as the blood supply for a free jejunal graft. If a long segment of native proximal esophagus is available, this resection of a portion of the clavicle, first rib, and manubrium may not be necessary because bolus transport into the thorax is facilitated by the normal contracting proximal esophagus. We have used the subcutaneous route only in extreme circumstances and as a last resort.

Remedial Surgery After Colonic Interposition

Patients who present with an intact but nonfunctional colon interposition pose difficult and challenging problems for the surgeon. In our experience, a poor result following colon interposition is usually caused by delayed gastric emptying of a retained stomach or graft tortuosity and redundancy. The creative use of a composite graft often can salvage the situation with an exceptionally good outcome. Usually enough proximal colon graft can be preserved to allow the placement of a jejunal graft between it and the antral portion of the stomach. The distal, dilated, redundant colon and proximal stomach are resected. Care must be taken not to interrupt the vascular pedicle to the colon graft. A longitudinal segment of the antimesenteric wall of the retained proximal colon is removed and the two sides of the colon rejoined over a 60 F bougie. This reduces the diameter of the proximal colon and turns it into an inert tube leading to a more active jejunal segment. We have performed four such remedial reconstructions and have found the resultant function to be surprisingly good (Fig. 15-4).

In summary, our preferred method of esophageal replacement after esophagectomy for benign disease, in patients fit to undergo such a procedure, is a vagal-spar-

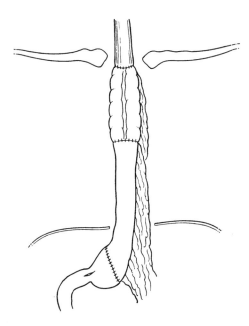

Fig. 15-4 Schematic drawing of a composite graft used to salvage patients presenting with an existing nonfunctional colon interposition. In most situations the size of the retained proximal colon is reduced by a coloplasty.

ing esophagectomy with colon interposition, with the colon anastomosed to the intact stomach. If the vagus nerves have been previously compromised or cannot be preserved during the procedure, a proximal two thirds gastrectomy is performed. If the colon is unsuitable for use as an esophageal substitute, or if the patient is elderly or infirm, the stomach is used. Only if both of these organs are unsuitable or unavailable is consideration given to using the jejunum, either as a transposition or as a free graft.

SURGICAL OUTCOME

In our series of 87 patients who underwent esophageal reconstruction for benign disease, two died in the hospital, resulting in a hospital mortality of 2%. Both died from sepsis with multiple organ failure. Graft necrosis occurred in two patients (2%), both with colon interpositions. One resulted in a hospital mortality and the other had an ischemic colon graft removed with subsequent reconstruction using a gastric interposition. A leak at one of the anastomotic sites occurred in five patients (6%). The most commonly affected anastomosis was the esophagocolostomy (Table 15-3). Of the six patients who required dilation after surgery, four had colon interpositions and two had gastric pull-ups. Only one patient had persistent dysphagia after a gastric interposition and has required intermittent dilations.

The median hospital stay was 17 days (range, 7 to 216 days). From the patient's perspective, it took a median of 2 weeks to fully recover (range, 1 to 96 weeks).

Table 15-3 Anastomotic leaks

Site	Total	No. of Leaks	%	Postoperative Day	Outcome
Esophagocolonic	71	3	4.2	4, 12, 28	Healed conservatively
					Died (sepsis)
					Healed conservatively with stenosis, reanastomosed successfully at 27 months
Cologastric	67	1	1.5	7	Healed conservatively
Esophagogastric	4	1	25	10	Healed conservatively

Table 15-4 Categories assessed by questionnaire

Recovery	Ingestion	Annoyances Related to Alimentation	Overall Satisfaction
Hospital stay	Number of meals/day	Dumping	Relief of symptoms
Recovery time	Meal capacity	Nausea	Outcome of surgery
	Diet restraints	Bloating	Risk/benefit assessment
	Last to finish	Frequent stools	
	Early satiety	Nocturnal regurgitation	
	Require liquids	Gurgling	
	Slow transit	Bad breath	
	Odynophagia		
	Choking		

Of the 87 patients who underwent esophageal reconstruction, 40 answered a postoperative questionnaire obtained by telephone interview. The questionnaire focused on recovery time, ability to ingest, annoyances related to alimentation, and overall patient satisfaction with the outcome of surgery (Table 15-4). The median follow-up period was 4 years (range, 2 months to 17 years). The remaining patients were unable to be contacted despite several attempts. Eighty-five percent of patients reported on the enjoyment of three meals a day without difficulty, while only 2% and 13% were limited to one or two meals, respectively. Fifty-three percent had the capacity to eat a steak dinner at one sitting, while 32% were limited to meals the size of an airline meal and 15% to a snack. Seventy-five percent of patients had the pleasure of an unrestricted diet. The process of ingestion was slower after esophageal replacement in that 62% of the patients were the last to finish in a group meal. Minor inconveniences in the patient's ability to ingest included the requirement for liquid in 32%, a sensation of slow transit in 25%, and choking in 2%. Some patients gained and others lost weight after the operation. Overall, the median change in weight was a gain of 10 pounds (range, −53 to +70 pounds).

Annoyances related to alimentation after esophageal replacement and reconstruction of the foregut are shown in Table 15-5. With the exception of gurgling,

Table 15-5 Annoyances related to alimentation after esophageal replacement in 40 patients

Complaints	%
Nausea	24
Bad breath	22
Nocturnal regurgitation	20
Bloating	12
Dumping	7
Frequent stools	5
Gurgling	2

bad breath, and nocturnal regurgitation in some patients, these complaints were present before surgery and persisted after reconstruction. The most bothersome symptom was nocturnal regurgitation and was alleviated by elevation of the head of the bed. All annoyances tended to abate with time.

Ninety-eight percent of patients judged that the operation had cured (25%) or improved (73%) their preoperative symptoms. Ninety-three percent were satisfied with the outcome of the operation. When asked to assess the overall risk or benefit of the procedure, 90% stated that, if faced with the decision again, they would choose to undergo the procedure again.

CONCLUSION

The observation that esophageal replacement and foregut reconstruction for benign disease can be performed with only a 2% mortality and minimal morbidity is encouraging to patients who are crippled from end-stage disease, previously failed surgery, or esophageal trauma. The continuation of slow, anxious, and socially restricted alimentation or maintenance of nutrition by enteral or parenteral means is unnecessary. The patient should be referred to a unit skilled in the evaluation of foregut function and the performance of esophageal replacement surgery. Despite the fact that some subtle preoperative symptoms of foregut dysfunction may persist after surgery, the overall outcome is generally judged to be satisfactory. Indeed, a patient can reenter society and live a normal and fulfilled life after remedial surgery. Long-term esophageal replacement for severe end-stage benign disease can be accomplished with low mortality, restoration of the pleasure of eating, and is viewed by the patient to be highly successful. Prolonged attempts at medical management of patients with severe derangements of esophageal structure and function are not warranted.

REFERENCES

1. DeMeester TR, Johansson K-E, Franze I, et al. Indications, surgical technique, and long-term functional results of colon interposition or bypass. Ann Surg 208:460-474, 1988.

2. Orringer MB, Sloan H. Esophagectomy without thoracotomy. J Thorac Cardiovasc Surg 76:643-654, 1978.
3. Holscher AH, Voit H, Buttermann G, et al. Function of the intrathoracic stomach as an esophageal replacement. World J Surg 12:835-844, 1988.
4. Orringer MB, Stirling MC. Cervical esophagogastric anastomosis for benign disease. J Thorac Cardiovasc Surg 96:887-893, 1988.
5. Belsey R. Reconstruction of the oesophagus. Ann R Coll Surg Engl 65:360-364, 1983.
6. Isolauri J, Helin H, Markkula H. Colon interposition for esophageal disease: Histologic findings of colonic mucosa after a follow-up of 5 months to 15 years. Am J Gastroenterol 86:277-280, 1991.
7. Engel JJ, Spellberg MA. Complications of vagotomy. Am J Gastroenterol 70:55-60, 1978.
8. Akiyama H, Tsurumaru M, Ono Y, et al. Esophagectomy without thoracotomy with vagal preservation. J Am Coll Surg 178:83-85, 1994.
9. Kelling G. Oesophagoplastik mit Hilfe des Querkolon. Zentralblatt Chir 38:1209-1212, 1911.
10. Vulliet H. De l'oesophagoplastie et des diverses modifications. Semaine Med 31:529-534, 1911.

16

Antroduodenal Motility in Foregut Disease

Johannes Heimbucher, M.D. • *Manfred P. Ritter, M.D.*
Hartmut Thomas, M.D.

Antroduodenal motility disorders contribute to several foregut pathologies, such as gastroesophageal reflux disease (GERD)[1-8] and peptic ulcer disease.[9-11] Delayed gastric emptying resulting from abnormal antral and/or duodenal motility patterns may cause an increase of acid gastroesophageal reflux[12] and stimulation of acid secretion with subsequent pH decrease of gastric contents.[13-16] Furthermore, duodenal juice, consisting of bile acids and pancreatic secretions, may cause gastric mucosal damage.[17-19] The clearance of duodenal juice from the stomach is a function of antroduodenal motility. Antroduodenal motility may therefore influence both the quantity and quality of refluxed material. Delay of gastric emptying and increased acid secretion may therefore play a part in the pathogenesis of peptic ulcer disease.[20-22] Rapid gastric emptying has been described in patients with duodenal ulcers[10] and dumping syndromes.[23] Finally, there is evidence that motility disorders play a major role in the irritable bowel syndrome.[24-26] During the last decade, the number of laboratories performing antroduodenal motility studies has grown, but the method still lacks a standardized technique and protocol.[27-29] Consequently, other techniques such as scintigraphic gastric-emptying or *o*-diisopropyl iminodiacetic acid (DISIDA) scan still have a higher clinical impact compared to antroduodenal motility.[13,30] Although these methods are inexpensive and noninvasive, they have the disadvantage of an assessment during a very short study period. The accuracy of these studies is not consistent because of the number of different protocols (liquid, solid, or mixed meals; upright or supine position; variance of detection systems) and the unphysiologic conditions for the patient during the study period.

The radionuclide test provides information about the consequences of disturbed motility, whereas antroduodenal manometry may help to recognize the pathophysiologic background. The value of antroduodenal motility studies has increased with the introduction of ambulatory motility devices providing new insights into antroduodenal motor activity. This chapter provides a description of normal antroduodenal motility patterns and the technique and protocol for antroduodenal motility studies at the University of Southern California. The analysis of data with a focus on specific circadian parameters will be explained, and a brief overview of results obtained from both symptom-free subjects and patients will be presented.

PHYSIOLOGY

The motor function of the stomach includes reception and storage of food, mixing of solid particles with saliva and gastric secretions, discrimination between solids and liquids, recognition of fat and protein contents, and the delivery of chyme through the pylorus into the duodenum at an appropriate rate for digestion and absorption.[31-33] Duodenal motor activity affects gastric emptying by changing the resistance to orthograde transpyloric flow and by retrograde activity that occurs during both postprandial and interdigestive states. The motor activity is regulated by electromechanical properties of the gastric and duodenal smooth muscle,[32,34] intestinal nerve plexuses, and intrinsic (myenteric plexus) and extrinsic (vagus, sympathic system) nerves.[35,36] Hormones, reacting on the consistency and size of a meal, nutrient content, acidity, and osmolality also modulate gastric and duodenal motor activity.[37,38] Receptors involved in that mechanism are located in the distal esophagus and in the upper small bowel. The stomach is anatomically divided into the fundus, corpus, and antrum. The motor functions, however, differ from the anatomic structures. The proximal stomach, including the fundus and approximately the upper third of the corpus, serves as a reservoir.[39,40] The main feature of this area is receptive relaxation and exhibits low amplitude tonic contractions. These contractions create a pressure gradient between the whole stomach and the duodenum promoting the emptying of liquids. The distal stomach, including the lower part of the corpus and antrum, mixes and compresses food particles and delivers chyme into the duodenum.[41] The three muscle layers of the stomach have an increasing thickness aborally and from the greater to the lesser curve.[42] The duodenum consists of the bulb, which produces coordinating contractions with the antral pump. The electrical activity of the antral contractions is generated from an area in the corpus along the greater curvature, which is considered to be the gastric pacemaker. The pacemaker propagates electrical activity circumferentially and aborally toward the duodenum. The frequency of the electrical potential activity in the stomach is three cycles per minute. This cycle is permanently present, but is not always associated with a gastric contraction. Contractions of a smooth muscle fiber are triggered by action potentials, which show an increased plateau potential.[32]

NORMAL ANTRODUODENAL MOTILITY

Mechanical activity of the antroduodenal region shows different patterns during either fasting or the fed state.[43-46] The fasting state exhibits a cyclical pattern called the migrating motor complex[47] or interdigestive myoelectric complex (interdigestive motility cycle [IMC]), consisting of three different degrees of activity, called phases (Fig. 16-1).

Phase 1 is a period of quiescence with almost no activity. It is the longest phase, lasting 45 to 60 minutes. Phase 2 shows intermittent contractions (frequency of 1

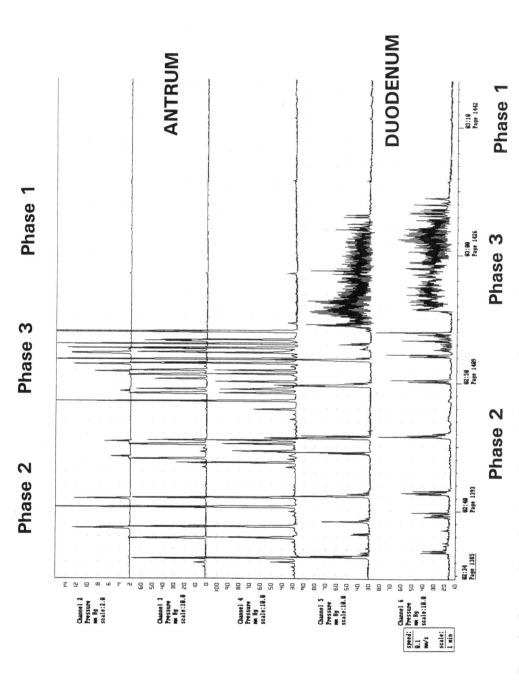

Fig. 16-1 Example of a normal interdigestive motility cycle. The upper three channels represent the duodenal activity, the lower two channels represent the antral activity. Note the increasing amplitude and frequency of antral contractions during phase 2. In this example phase 3 lasts 5 minutes in the antrum and 8 minutes in the duodenum.

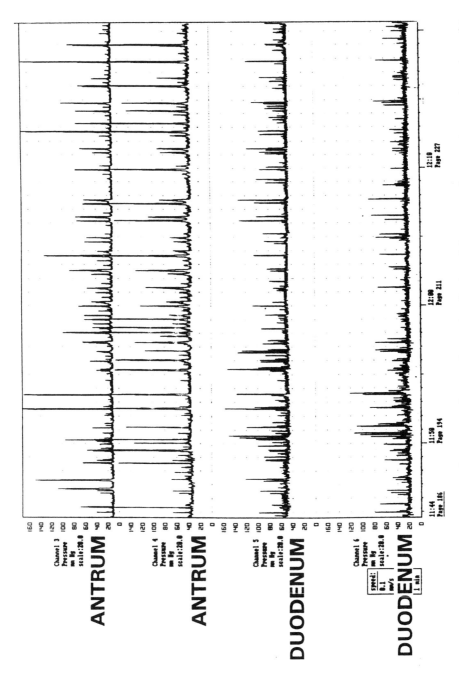

Fig. 16-2 Example of a normal fed pattern. There are no distinct phases. Amplitude and frequency of contractions are irregular and increased.

to 2 per minute in the antrum, 2 to 5 per minute in the duodenum), which increase in frequency and amplitude over a period of 30 minutes. Phase 3 consists of a crescendo of the most dynamic activity with 2.5 to 3.5 antral contractions and 8 to 12 duodenal contractions per minute. This feature lasts for 5 to 10 minutes and is termed the migrating motor complex (MMC). Some authors describe the brief transition period between the maximal activity of phase 3 and the quiescence of phase 1 as phase 4.[48] One complete cycle (IMC) of all three phases lasts 90 to 120 minutes. The IMC migrates from the stomach and propagates down to the entire small intestine.[48] Movement of any remaining gastric contents after the fed pattern is completed strongly correlates with the motility phases. During phase 1 there is almost no movement, during phase 2 there is more mixing of contents than propulsion. Phase 3 provides the aboral propulsion of large undigestible contents.[32] This cyclical activity repeats itself until it is disrupted by ingestion of food.

The typical fed pattern motility consists of intermittent contractions similar to phase 2[49] (Fig. 16-2). The duration of the postprandial activity depends on the food characteristics, such as quantity or fat and protein content.[45,50] Antroduodenal motility shows circadian changes.

INDICATIONS FOR ANTRODUODENAL MOTILITY STUDIES

Antroduodenal motility studies are used to evaluate patients who have upper gastrointestinal symptoms but negative radiologic and endoscopic investigations. Such symptoms include early satiety, prolonged postprandial discomfort, bloating, abdominal distention, nausea, vomiting, diarrhea, cramping, and maldigestion. These symptoms are nonspecific and may reflect either gastric disorders or disturbances in other intestinal regions or combinations of different dysfunctions involving motor activity in specific regions, secretion, and absorptive function. A precise diagnosis of gut dysmotility can rarely be made on a clinical basis alone, especially in terms of identifying the regions involved. Therefore, application of a relevant diagnostic test is desirable. The indication for the study should be based on the intensity and chronicity of symptoms.[28,51] In patients with established pathology, the result of an antroduodenal motility study may help to choose the most appropriate therapeutic alternative, especially by identification of the region involved in the motility disorder. Significance of motor abnormalities should be carefully weighted and interpreted in comparison to other studies (i.e., scintigraphic gastric emptying). Antroduodenal motility studies may also be used to monitor the progress of a motor disorder and to certify the effect of pharmacologic therapy.[52]

TECHNIQUE

Since stationary systems have a number of drawbacks and limitations for antroduodenal motility studies, only the ambulatory technique with electronic strain gauge transducers is described. Catheters are available in multiple different shapes. It is important that there is only a short distance between the antral transducers and that the apparatus is smooth and elastic for the patient's comfort. We use a five-channel solid-state catheter (Konigsberg Instruments, Pasadena, Calif.) with three transducers oriented 120 degrees to each other, spaced at 2 cm distances for antral measurement, and two transducers 10 cm apart for duodenal measurements. This catheter is connected to a portable data logger with 4 megabyte memory (Microdigitrapper; Synectics Medical, Dallas, Tex.) as data storage. Data are processed with an IBM AT personal computer using specifically designed software (Multigram; Gastrosoft, Inc., Irving, Tex.).

PROTOCOL

All potentially interfering drugs must be discontinued at least 48 hours prior to the examination. After an overnight fast, the motility catheter is passed transnasally down the esophagus through the stomach and into the duodenum. Under fluoroscopic guidance, the final position of the catheter is achieved, with the most orad pressure sensor sited 5 cm proximal to the pylorus. When correctly positioned, three pressure sensors are recording antral pressure changes and two are recording duodenal pressure changes in the mid-descending and fourth part of the duodenum, respectively (Fig. 16-3). The slack in the catheter is taken up so that it lies snugly against the lesser curve of the stomach. This position is chosen because it detects antral contractions as well as the migration of contractions through the pyloric region and the contractions of the duodenum. Data collected in this setup allow for a very precise and comprehensive image of the present antroduodenal motility pattern. The study period is 24 hours. The patient should perform his or her normal daily activities during the investigation but smokers are encouraged to

A

B

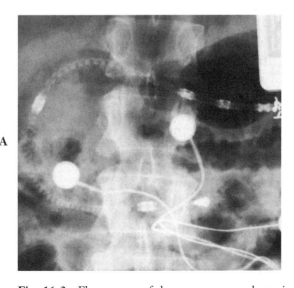
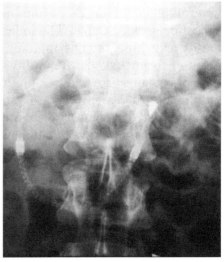

Fig. 16-3 Fluoroscopy of the manometry catheter in place. There are three sensors spaced 2 cm apart in the antrum and two sensors spaced 10 cm apart in the duodenum.

avoid smoking. The patient is instructed to eat at set times only (lunch, dinner, and breakfast) as indicated in a diary. This provides adequate information of both fasting- and fed-state motility patterns. All symptoms occurring during the study period should also be indicated in this diary to allow for a correlation of symptoms with motility features. The subject is allowed to return home with the manometry probe in position and connected to the microdigitrapper, which stores all data over the full study period.

ANALYSIS

A specifically designed software program that analyzes antroduodenal motility data (Multigram) is able to quantify wave activity and recognize several motility patterns. A pressure change greater than 9 mm Hg of 1- to 10-second duration is recognized as a contraction. The definition of the different fasting phases is variable and is determined by the frequency of contractions and the minimum duration of the phase. Phase 1 is recognized when contractions in the antrum are less than one per minute and are longer than 10 minutes in duration; phase 2 is when there are one to two contractions per minute lasting longer than 10 minutes in duration; and phase 3 is when there are three to five contractions per minute of longer than 2 minutes' duration. The antral analysis is performed using the best of the three channels only. Because of the wide lumen of the antral region, not every contraction may be recorded from each channel. For the duodenal analysis we require less than one contraction per minute and longer than 10 minutes in duration for phase 1, one to six contractions per minute and longer than 10 minutes in duration for phase 2, and seven to 12 contractions per minute and longer than 3 minutes in duration for phase 3. The fed pattern is identified by the typical change from the fasting pattern, which occurs after the beginning of the meal, and in some individuals even shortly before the meal is begun. The analysis by calculation of contraction characteristics and a motility index is performed for a 2-hour period or until the next phase 3 occurs. In the analysis summary the program offers a characterization of the IMC, indicating the detected phase 3, the order of its propagation, the velocity of propagation, its motility index, and the duration and contraction frequency of each previous phase. The fed pattern is characterized by the number of contractions recorded in each channel, the frequency, mean amplitude and duration of contractions, and a motility index. A similar contraction analysis is performed for the whole study period. Furthermore, the program features a graphic display of the phases during the study with indication of meals and supine periods. Although the software is convenient to use, most of the results are at the present time more useful for the clinical investigator than of help to the clinician. Supplementary information with clinical relevance may be achieved by performing an additional visual and manual analysis of the record and by calculating parameters that are not included in the current version of the program. Visual reading of the tracings requires dedication and some experience to avoid overenthusiastic interpretation of supposed abnormalities. The new parameters used help to retrieve the information of an extended study period. Atypical motility features that occur during symptomatic

Table 16-1   Normal values of antroduodenal motility

	Antrum	Duodenum
Contractions		
Phase 2		
Motility index/min	3-5	4-6
Frequency/min	1-1.5	1.5-4.5
Mean duration	1.7-3.5	1.5-3
Mean amplitude	10-25	10-20
Phase 3		
Motility index/min	4-10	4-10
Frequency/min	2.5-4	7-14
Mean duration	1.5-4	1.3-3
Mean amplitude mm Hg	40-100	10-40
Fed pattern		
Motility index	3-6	2.5-4.8
Frequency	0.5-3	0.5-2.7
Mean duration	2-3.6	2-3.8
Mean amplitude	15-35	13-28
IMC characteristics		
Total activity (%)		
Phase 1*	15-30	10-25
Phase 2*	20-50	40-60
Phase 3*	3-5	3-5
Fed pattern*	5-20	5-20
Complete IMCs		
Total 24-hour study	4-8	4-10
Mean duration	80-120	80-140
Phase 1%	30-45	10-35
Phase 2%	20-50	50-80
Phase 3%	3-5	3-6
Daytime	1-3	1-3
Mean duration	75-110	60-110
Phase 1%	30-45	10-35
Phase 2%	20-50	50-80
Phase 3%	3-5	3-6
Nighttime	2-4	3-5
Mean duration	80-140	80-140
Phase 1%	40-60	15-40
Phase 2%	15-40	50-85
Phase 3%	3-5	3-5
Coordination		
Abnormal sequences*	<10%	<10%
Antroduodenal linkage*	>80%	>80%
Migration velocity (cm/sec)	0.2-0.45	0.15-0.4
Orthograde migration	>90%	>80%
Cluster activity*	1-8	1-8
Fed pattern		
Time to onset (min)	0-8	−2-6
Duration	60-180	60-180
Motility index	3-6	2.5-4.8

IMC = Interdigestive motility cycle.
*Parameters assessed by manual analysis only.

periods may be recognized more sensitively when the original tracing is reviewed. Technical problems, such as displacement of the probe or motion artifacts, are identified by the software, which recognizes typical gastric or duodenal patterns only. The fed pattern should be analyzed together with the clinical presentation of the patient. Postprandial activity is expressed by a motility index (MI), which incorporates frequency and amplitude of contractions for 2 hours after ingestion of a meal. MI is calculated for 15-minute intervals and as a total 2-hour index. No interdigestive pattern may appear in patients with severe delay of gastric emptying during the daytime study period because residual gastric contents may be present at the beginning of each meal. Theoretically, a continuous-fasting pattern may also result from poor gastric emptying since incomplete nutrient delivery into the duodenum may fail to trigger the conversion to a fed pattern. Parameters calculated by the computerized analysis and manually assessed data are listed in Table 16-1.

RESULTS
Normal Values for Antroduodenal Motility Studies

Using the described protocol and technique, results were obtained for symptom-free subjects (n = 30) as listed in Table 16-1. There are four different analyses: (1) parameters describing the single contractions during phase 2, phase 3, and the fed pattern; (2) parameters describing the IMC characteristics; (3) parameters describing antroduodenal coordination; and (4) parameters describing the fed pattern. All parameters of the first two sections and most parameters of the third and fourth were analyzed individually for antral and duodenal activity as well as total time, daytime, and nighttime. Note particularly the markedly different results of IMC parameters for daytime and nighttime studies.

Abnormal Fasting Antroduodenal Motility Features
Antral Hypomotility

A hypomotility pattern demonstrates a decrease of both frequency and amplitude of contractions, which is found in the interdigestive period as well as during the fed state. A shortening or complete absence of activity in phases 2 or 3 and the fed pattern may also be found (Fig. 16-4). Parameters that indicate antral hypomotility are decreased amplitude and duration of single contractions, duration of phases (prolonged phase 1, shortened phases 2 and 3), duration and motility index of fed pattern, and number of complete IMCs. Hypomotile states are seen in myopathic diseases (scleroderma and other collagen vascular diseases, muscular dystrophies, and amyloidosis),[53-55] neuropathic diseases (diabetes mellitus, multiple sclerosis), and spinal cord injury with consequent extrinsic nerve dysfunction.[56-58] Symptomatic patients following foregut surgery often present with antroduodenal motility disorders similar to neurogenic changes. After vagotomy the response to a meal is often reduced.[56,59-61] We obtained also a reduced number of antral phase 3 during the fasting state in postvagotomy patients. The 24-hour study has shown that diabetic patients with symptoms of gastroparesis may develop close to normal patterns during the supine period. This may be due to a prolonged hypomotile fed

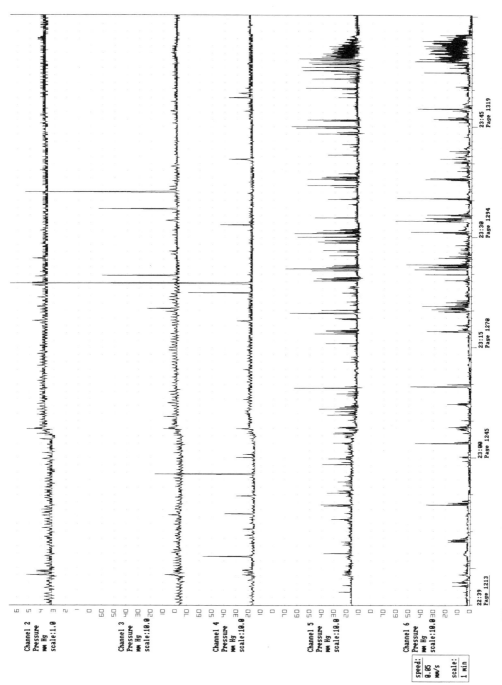

Fig. 16-4   Antral hypomotility. Only a few typical antral contractions occur during phase 2 and phase 3.

pattern during the daytime. Patients with scleroderma exhibit a hypomotile pattern in both the antrum and duodenum during fasting and the fed period. Antral and/or duodenal hypomotility resulting in delayed gastric emptying and stasis of gastric secretions may generate additional foregut pathology.

Increased Phasic Activity

Recurring episodes of intense regular, often simultaneous, contractions followed by periods of rest have been observed proximal to an obstruction.[62,63] The episodes of these contractions are often associated with crampy abdominal pain (Fig. 16-5). Another sign of pathologic increased motor activity are bursts of non-propagating pressure waves lasting for up to 30 minutes. They occur only at one level without association to activity at an adjacent level (segmental activity). Parameters that indicate increased phasic activity are increased amplitude and duration of single contractions, increased duration of phases (prolonged phase 3), increased duration and motility index of the fed pattern, and propagation velocity of single contractions. Conditions in this category are neurogenic disorders, intoxications, and endocrine dysfunctions such as hyperthyroidism.[64] Antral hypermotility in pyloric and duodenal ulcer patients may be caused by organic stenosis or an increased vagal tone.

Disturbed Antroduodenal Coordination

The main features of incoordination are a shortened or missing phase 3, abnormal migration of phase 3, and failure of the fed pattern with continuous fasting motility (Fig. 16-6). Parameters that indicate antroduodenal incoordination are abnormal sequence of phases, abnormal number of complete IMCs, and abnormal propagation velocity and direction of phase 3. Neurogenic diseases and patients with diabetes mellitus demonstrate these patterns.[56,65-67] A recent study of antroduodenal motility features in patients following cholecystectomy showed both a hypomotile pattern and a disordered coordination, which was associated with increased duodenogastric reflux in symptomatic patients.[68,69] Unfortunately, it was not established whether the motility disorder was present before surgery. Antroduodenal and more extensive motility disorders, including the biliary system, might be a cofactor in the pathogenesis of gallstone disease.[70]

Duodenal Abnormalities

Isolated duodenal motility disorders are rarely reported.[71,72] A typical finding is a clustering of contractions, a group of strong regular contractions with an elevated baseline with more than 3 minutes of quiescence beforehand and afterwards. Another frequent feature is the increased number of IMCs or the appearance of additional phase 3–like activity caused by the duodenal pacemaker (Fig. 16-7). These abnormalities may be present in neurogenic diseases and the irritable bowel syndrome. *Text continued on p. 228.*

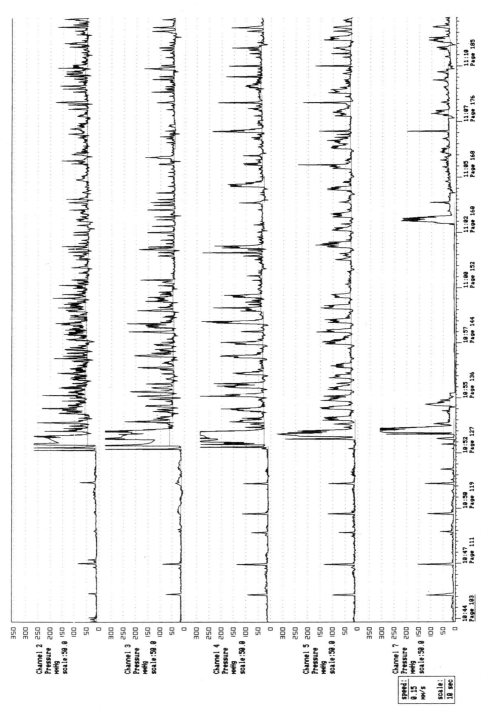

Fig. 16-5   Paroxysmal antral hypermotility. Frequent contractions with high amplitude, which were coincident with crampy abdominal pain in this example.

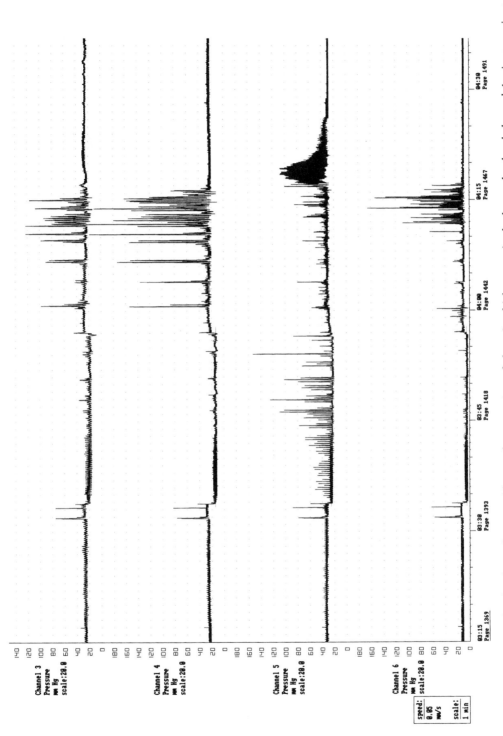

Fig. 16-6 Disturbed antroduodenal coordination. Abnormal propagation of phase 3, which occurs in the lower duodenal channel 4 minutes prior to phase 3 activity in the upper duodenal channel.

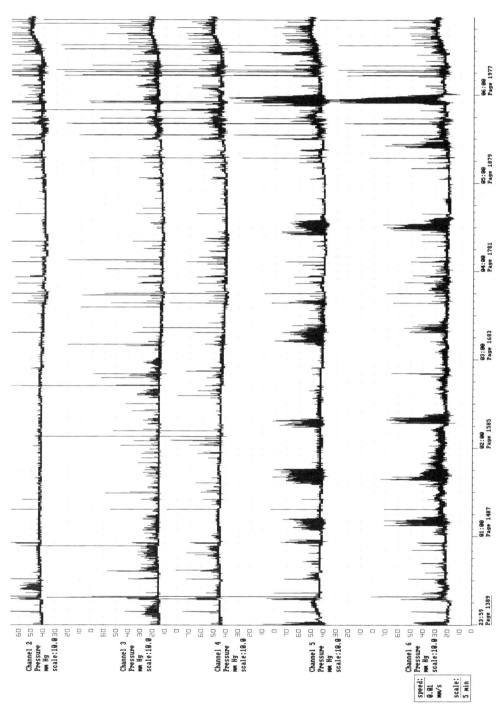

Fig. 16-7 Duodenal abnormality. Additional phase 3–like activity in the duodenal channels occurring in 30- to 60-minute intervals. This phenomenon indicates secondary pacemaker activity, which was associated with symptoms of dumping in this patient.

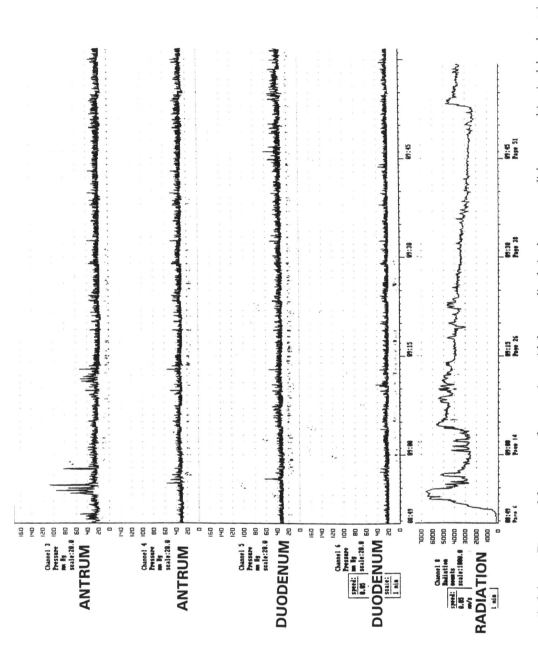

Fig. 16-8   Hypomotile fed state. Decreased frequency of contractions with low amplitude in the postprandial state resulting in delayed gastric empty-ing, which was documented by a synchronous scintigraphic gastric-emptying study.

Abnormal Postprandial Antroduodenal Motility Features

During the fed state, all types of abnormal patterns similar to the fasting pattern may occur. Since there is no basic pattern such as the IMC, the precise quantification of any abnormality is more difficult. Abnormally low motility indices due to a reduced number of contractions as well as a low amplitude, absent or incomplete conversion from the interdigestive pattern, delayed onset of the fed pattern, and premature return to the interdigestive pattern (Fig. 16-8) may be documented.

Before an antroduodenal motility study is considered to be abnormal, there should be multiple parameters outside the normal range. Furthermore, symptoms during specific periods of abnormal motility should be present. The presence of abnormal results in only a few of the many possible parameters should lead to a guarded interpretation, since there is a wide variation of the normal pattern. Parameters that integrate the whole study period, such as total activity, number of complete IMCs, and coordinative values, have shown to be most sensitive and correlate with abnormal results in complementary tests such as scintigraphic gastric emptying and gastric pH-metry. Antral and duodenal activity should be defined separately.

LIMITATIONS

The invasiveness of an antroduodenal manometry study (transnasal intubation, x-ray) and some technical difficulties, such as intubating the pylorus for correct placement of the probe, have handicapped its routine use. However, modern specially shaped catheters with smooth tips and smooth upper parts that lie in the nasopharyngeal area and a more rigid middle segment are easier to pass through the pylorus and more convenient for the patient. With some experience and technical skill, the placement can be completed within 2 to 5 minutes. A standard for analysis of antroduodenal motility data has not been established, and there are no specific pathologic patterns leading to a precise diagnosis. The highly variable motor patterns require careful correlation with symptoms and correlation with other tests. This will also help to determine whether present motor abnormalities are primary changes or secondary to other organic or functional pathology. Frequently the observed abnormality is not related to symptoms and a single study does not reveal that a dysfunction is permanent or transient. Therefore, prolonged (longer than 24 hours) or repeated antroduodenal motility studies may be helpful in special cases. Nasogastric duodenal intubation itself may have an influence on the motility.[73,74] Migration of the catheter during the study may be identified by typical antral and duodenal patterns. Close spacing of antral sensors is important to detect antral contractions as well as migration of the catheter.

CLINICAL IMPLICATIONS AND THERAPEUTIC IMPACT OF ANTRODUODENAL MOTILITY STUDIES

Assessment of gastric motor function includes multiple tests such as scintigraphic gastric emptying, ultrasonography, and electrogastrography. However, only

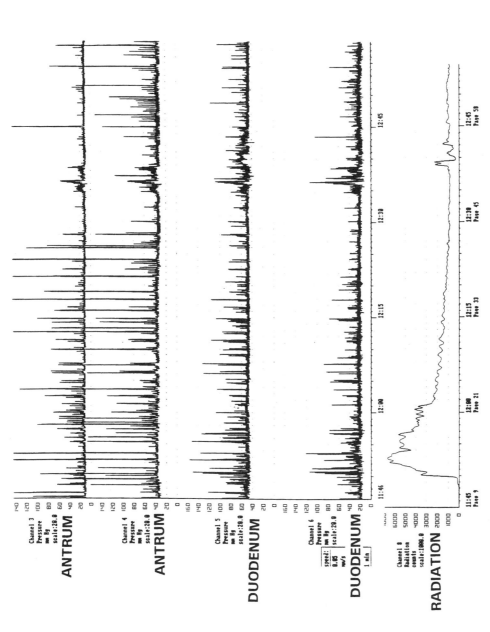

Fig. 16-9 Combined antroduodenal manometry and scintigraphic gastric-emptying study using an ambulatory device. There is a typical fed pattern resulting in normal gastric emptying during the first hour of the study.

manometric studies provide a detailed information of the motility in the antroduodenal region. Antroduodenal motility studies confirm the presence of a pathologic pattern in severe cases and contribute to the diagnosis in borderline cases. A myopathic or neuropathic hypomotile or hypermotile pattern of motility disorder may be determined. Furthermore, the study demonstrates whether the motility disorder occurs throughout the whole antroduodenal complex or is restricted to the stomach or rarely the duodenum. The identification of isolated gastric hypomotility will prompt the use of prokinetic medication or the need for near total gastrectomy in severe cases of gastroparesis. Documentation of a myopathic process is important because prokinetics are not effective in such cases.[27,75]

FUTURE PERSPECTIVES

The value of less invasive methods to study gastric motor function, such as EGG, ultrasonography, and scintigraphy, may be improved by performing such studies simultaneously with antroduodenal manometry (Fig. 16-9). The postprandial state is the most important period to be studied (Fig. 16-8). A more comprehensive image of gastric motor function may be achieved by complementary studies with the Barostat, which monitors the fundic tone. The use of a sleeve sensor in the manometry probe may clarify the role of pyloric contractions. Detection of catheter migration during the study will be more precise by including potential difference electrodes in the probe. All additional aspects to be assessed require more sophisticated probes, which are currently being developed as are extended receiving and storage capacities of the electronic devices. The computerized analysis of motility data also needs improvement and validation by more and extended studies of normal subjects. A major goal will be a simplification and concentration on data of clinical relevance.

CONCLUSION

Gastrointestinal motility disorders constitute a major segment of digestive disease. Therefore, measurement of gut motor activity should be a desired goal. Antroduodenal manometry is potentially helpful in the diagnostic evaluation of patients presenting with upper gastrointestinal symptoms without demonstrable anatomic alteration as evidenced by conventional diagnostic evaluation. Antroduodenal motility may help to localize the affected region of the gut, as well as to monitor the evolution of the motor disorder, and to determine the effect of pharmacologic treatment. Measurement of antroduodenal motility has matured with new methodologic developments. It has proved its value to an extent that its application to clinical gastroenterology in carefully selected cases is now appropriate and timely, especially in relationship to the new prokinetic drugs.

REFERENCES

1. DeMeester TR, Johnson LF, Joseph GJ, Toscano MS, Hall AW, Skinner DB. Patterns of gastroesophageal reflux in health and disease. Ann Surg 184:459-470, 1976.

2. Hsu WH, Chien KY, DeMeester TR, Skinner DB. Studies of esophageal manometry, esophageal pH monitoring, and gastric emptying scan in gastroesophageal reflux patients. J Surg Assoc 17: 335-345, 1984.

3. Schwizer W, Hinder RA, DeMeester TR. Does delayed gastric emptying contribute to gastroesophageal reflux disease? Am J Surg 157:74-81, 1989.

4. Pope CE. Is LES enough? Gastroenterology 71:328-329, 1976.

5. Gowen GF. Spontaneous enterogastric reflux gastritis and esophagitis. Ann Surg 201:170-175, 1985.

6. Little AG, DeMeester TR, Rezai-Zadeh K, Skinner DB. Abnormal gastric emptying in patients with gastroesophageal reflux. Surg Forum 28:347-348, 1977.

7. Hinder RA, Stein HJ, Bremner CG, DeMeester TR. Relationship of a satisfactory outcome to normalization of delayed gastric emptying after Nissen fundoplication. Ann Surg 210:458-465, 1989.

8. McCallum RW, Berkowitz DM, Lerner E. Gastric emptying in patients with gastroesophageal reflux. Gastroenterology 80:285-291, 1981.

9. Stanghellini V, Ghidini C, Maccarini MR, Paparo GF, Corinaldesi R, Barbara L. Fasting and postprandial gastrointestinal motility in ulcer and non-ulcer dyspepsia. Gut 33:184-190, 1992.

10. Kerrigan DD, Read NW, Houghton LA, Taylor ME, Johnson AG. Disturbed gastroduodenal motility in patients with active and healed duodenal ulceration. Gastroenterology 100:892-900, 1991.

11. Morguelan B, Ippoliti A, Sturdevant R. Gastric emptying in patients with gastric ulcer. Gastroenterology 74:1070, 1978.

12. Samelson SL, Weiser HF, Bombeck T, Siewert JR, Ludtke FE, Hoelscher AH. A new concept in the surgical treatment of gastroesophageal reflux. Ann Surg 197:254-259, 1983.

13. Scarpignato C. Gastric emptying in gastroesophageal reflux disease and other functional esophageal disorders. In Scarpignato C, Galmiche JP, eds. Frontiers in Gastrointestinal Research, vol. 22. Functional Evaluation in Esophageal Disease. Basel: Karger, 1994, pp 223-259.

14. Barlow AP, DeMeester TR, Ball CS, Eypasch EP. The significance of the gastric secretory state in gastroesophageal reflux disease. Arch Surg 124:937-940, 1989.

15. Stein HJ, DeMeester TR, Hinder RA. Outpatient physiologic testing and surgical management of functional foregut disorders. Curr Probl Surg 24:418-555, 1992.

16. Stein HJ, Barlow AP, DeMeester TR, Hinder RA. Complications of gastroesophageal reflux disease: Role of the lower esophageal sphincter, esophageal acid and acid/alkaline exposure, and duodenogastric reflux. Ann Surg 216:35-43, 1992.

17. Little AG, Martinez EL, DeMeester TR, Blough RM, Skinner DB. Duodenogastric reflux and reflux esophagitis. Surgery 96:447-454, 1984.

18. Fuchs KH, DeMeester TR, Schwizer W, Albertucci M. Concomitant duodenogastric and gastroesophageal reflux: The role of twenty-four-hour gastric pH monitoring. In Siewert JR, Holscher AH, eds. Diseases of the Esophagus. New York: Springer-Verlag, 1987, pp 1073-1076.

19. Ritchie WP. Harmful effects of enterogastric reflux in the stomach. Probl Gen Surg 10:236-241, 1993.

20. Thompson DG, Ritchie HD, Wingate DL. Patterns of small intestinal motility in duodenal ulcer patients before and after vagotomy. Gut 23:51-58, 1982.

21. Williams NS, Grossman MI, Meyer JH. Abnormalities of gastric emptying of liquids in duodenal ulcer disease. Dig Dis Sci 31:943-952, 1986.

22. Hoeft SF, Yasui A, DeMeester TR, Hinder RA, Hagen JA, Bremner RM. Delayed gastric emptying favors development of gastric mucosal damage in duodenogastric reflux. Gastroenterology 102:A458, 1992.

23. Haynes S, Thomson JPS, Brown N. A study of the relationship between the rate of gastric emptying and the dumping syndrome. Br J Surg 60:307-308, 1973.

24. Kumar D, Wingate DL. The irritable bowel syndrome. A paroxysmal motor disorder. Lancet 2:973-977, 1985.

25. Kellow JE, Gill RC, Wingate DL. Prolonged ambulant recordings of small bowel motility demonstrate abnormalities in the irritable bowel syndrome. Gastroenterology 98:1208-1218, 1990.

26. Kumar D, Wingate DL. The irritable bowel syndrome: A profound motor disorder. Lancet 2:973-977, 1985.

27. Camilleri M. Study of human gastroduodenal motility: Applied physiology in clinical practice. Dig Dis Sci 38:785-794, 1993.

28. Mearin F, Malagelada JR. Gastrointestinal manometry: A practical tool or a research technique? J Clin Gastroenterol 16:281-291, 1993.

29. Quigley EMM, Donovan JP, Lane MJ, Gallagher TF. Antroduodenal manometry: Usefulness and limitations as an outpatient study. Dig Dis Sci 37:20-28, 1992.

30. Camilleri M, Zinsmeister AR, Greydanus MP, Brown ML, Proano M. Towards a less costly but accurate test of gastric emptying and small bowel transit. Dig Dis Sci 36:609-615, 1991.

31. Cannon WB, Lieb CW. The receptive relaxation of the stomach. Am J Physiol 29:267-272, 1911.

32. Kelly KA. Motility of the stomach and gastroduodenal junction. In Johnson LR, ed. Physiology of the Gastrointestinal Tract. New York: Raven Press, 1981, pp 393-410.

33. Jahnberg T. Gastric adaptative relaxation. Scand J Gastroenterol 12:1-6, 1977.

34. Weber J Jr, Kohatsu S. Pacemaker localization and electrical conduction patterns in the canine stomach. Gastroenterology 59:717-723, 1970.

35. Hall KE, El-Sharkawy TY, Diamant NE. Vagal control of migrating motor complex in the dog. Am J Physiol 243:G276-281, 1982.

36. Gleystenn JJ, Sarna SK, Myrvik AL. Canine cyclic motor activity of the stomach and small bowel: The vagus is not the governor. Gastroenterology 88:1926-1931, 1985.

37. Marik F, Code CF. Control of interdigestive myoelectric activity in dogs by the vagus nerves and pentagastrin. Gastroenterology 69:387-390, 1975.

38. Weisbrodt NW. The regulation of gastrointestinal motility. In Anuras S, ed. Motility Disorders of the Gastrointestinal Tract. New York: Raven Press, 1992, pp 27-48.

39. Meyer JH. Motility of the stomach and gastroduodenal junction. In Johnson LR, ed. Physiology of the Gastrointestinal Tract, 2nd ed. New York: Raven Press, 1987, pp 613-630.

40. Kelly KA. Gastric emptying of liquids and solids: Roles of proximal and distal stomach. Am J Physiol 239:G71-76, 1980.

41. Camilleri M, Malagelada JR, Brown ML, Becker G, Zinsmeister AR. Relationship between antral motility and gastric emptying in humans. Am J Physiol 12:G580-585, 1985.

42. Gabella G. Structure of muscles and nerves in the gastrointestinal tract. In Johnson LR, ed. Physiology of the Gastrointestinal Tract, 2nd ed. New York: Raven Press, 1987, pp 335-381.

43. Itoh Z, Aizawa I, Sekiguchi T. The interdigestive migrating complex and its significance in man. Clin Gastroenterol 11:497-521, 1982.

44. Keane FB, DiMagno EP, Malagelada JR. Duodenogastric reflux in humans: Its relationship to fasting antroduodenal motility and gastric, pancreatic, and biliary secretion. Gastroenterology 81:726-731, 1981.

45. Rees WDW, Go VLW, Malagelada JR. Antroduodenal motor response to solid-liquid and homogenized meals. Gastroenterology 76:1438-1442, 1979.

46. Houghton LA, Read NW, Heddle R, Maddern GJ, Downton J, Toouli J, Dent J. Motor activity of the gastric antrum, pylorus, and duodenum under fasted conditions and after a liquid meal. Gastroenterology 94:1276-1284, 1988.

47. Sarna SK. Cyclic motor activity: Migrating motor complex. Gastroenterology 89:894-913, 1985.

48. Szurszewski JH. A migrating electric complex of the canine small intestine. Am J Physiol 317:1757-1763, 1969.

49. Read NW, Al-Janabi MN, Edwards CA, Barber DC. Relationship between postprandial motor activity in human small intestine and the gastrointestinal transit of food. Gastroenterology 86:721-727, 1984.

50. Welch IM, Worlding J. The effect of ileal infusion of lipid on the motility pattern in humans after ingestion of a viscous non-nutrient meal. J Physiol 378:12P, 1986.

51. Costantini M, Crookes PF, Bremner RM, Hoeft SF, Afshin E, Peters JH, Bremner CG, De-Meester TR. Value of physiologic assessment of foregut symptoms in a surgical practice. Surgery 114:780-787, 1993.
52. Fraser RJ, Horowitz M, Maddox AF, Dent J. Postprandial antropyloroduodenal motility and gastric emptying in gastroparesis—Effects of cisapride. Gut 35:172-178, 1994.
53. Rees WDW, Leigh RJ, Christofides ND, Bloom SR, Turnberg LA. Interdigestive motor activity in patients with systemic sclerosis. Gastroenterology 83:575-580, 1982.
54. DiMarino A, Carlson G, Myers A, Schumacher R, Cohen S. Duodenal myoelectric activity in scleroderma. N Engl J Med 289:1220-1223, 1973.
55. Wald A, Kichler J, Mendelow H. Amyloidosis and chronic intestinal pseudoobstruction. Dig Dis Sci 26:462-465, 1981.
56. Malagelada JR, Rees WDW, Mazotta LG. Gastric motor abnormalities in diabetic and post-vagotomy gastroparesis: Effect of metoclopramide and benthanechol. Gastroenterology 78:286-293, 1980.
57. Nowak TV, Anuras S, Brown BT. Small intestinal motility in myotonic dystrophy patients. Gastroenterology 86:808-813, 1984.
58. Fealy RD, Szurszewski JH, Meritt JL, DiMagno EP. Effect of spinal cord transection on human gastrointestinal motility and gastric emptying. Gastroenterology 87:69-75, 1984.
59. Hinder RA, Bremner CG. Relative role of pyloroplasty size, truncal vagotomy and milk meal volume in canine gastric emptying. Am J Dig Dis 23:210-216, 1978.
60. Kelly KA, Code CF. Effect of transthoracic vagotomy of canine gastric electrical activity. Gastroenterology 57:51-59, 1969.
61. Wilbur BG, Kelly KA. Effect of proximal gastric, complete gastric, and truncal vagotomy on canine gastric electric activity, motility, and emptying. Ann Surg 178:295-301, 1973.
62. Summers RW, Anuras S, Green J. Jejunal manometry patterns in health, partial intestinal obstruction, and pseudoobstruction. Gastroenterology 85:1290-1300, 1983.
63. Camilleri M. Jejunal manometry in distal subacute mechanical obstruction: Significance of prolonged simultaneous contractions. Gut 30:468-475, 1989.
64. Miller L, Gorman C, Go V. Gut-thyroid interrelationships. Gastroenterology 75:901-908, 1978.
65. Feldman M, Scjiller LR. Disorders of gastrointestinal motility associated with diabetes mellitus. Ann Intern Med 98:378-384, 1983.
66. Camilleri M, Malagelada JR. Abnormal intestinal motility in diabetics with the gastroparesis syndrome. Eur J Clin Invest 14:420-427, 1984.
67. Summers RW, Karacis JJ, Anuras S. Pseudoobstruction syndrome in multiple sclerosis. J Gastrointest Motil 3:144-150, 1991.
68. Perdikis G, Wilson P, Hinder RA, Redmont E, Wetscher G, Neary P, Adrian T, Quigley E. Altered antroduodenal motility after cholecystectomy. Am J Surg 168:609-615, 1994.
69. Inoue K, Fuchigami A, Higashide S. Gallbladder sludge and stone formation in relation to contractile function after gastrectomy. Ann Surg 215:19-26, 1992.
70. Lujan-Mompean JA, Robles-Campos R, Parilla-Paricio P, Liron-Ruiz R, Torralba-Martinez JA, Cifuentes-Tebar J. Duodenogastric reflux in patients with biliary lithiasis before and after cholecystectomy. Surg Gynecol Obstet 176:116-118, 1993.
71. Camilleri M, Brown ML, Malagelada JR. Relationship between impaired gastric emptying and abnormal gastrointestinal motility. Gastroenterology 91:94-99, 1986.
72. Malagelada JR, Stanghellini V. Manometric evaluation of functional upper gut symptoms. Gastroenterology 88:1223-1231, 1985.
73. Camilleri M, Neri M. Motility disorders and stress. Dig Dis Sci 34:1777-1785, 1989.
74. Read NW, Al-Janabi MN, Bates TE, Barber DC. Effect of gastrointestinal intubation on the passage of a solid meal through the stomach and small intestine in humans. Gastroenterology 84:1568-1573, 1983.
75. Waters PF, DeMeester TR. Foregut motor disorders and their surgical management. Med Clin North Am 65:1235-1268, 1981.

Index